At an age when most people are considering retirement, Libby Wilson took up the challenge of a year's work in Sierra Leone. Having practised for forty years in the field of women's health, *Unexpected Always Happen* is an energetic account of a doctor's experience of Africa.

Life in one of the world's poorest countries was never going to be easy, but Dr. Wilson has produced an engaging travelogue on the ups and downs of life and death in West Africa. The dangers to health, the chaos and corruption of public life and the energy of the people in the face of adversity make a real and heartening story.

Unexpected Always Happen

Journal of a Doctor in Sierra-Leone

Libby Wilson

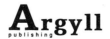

© Dr. Libby Wilson, 1995

First published in 1995 by
Argyll Publishing
Glendaruel
Argyll PA22 3AE
Scotland

The author has asserted her moral rights.

To preserve confidentiality, some names and places
have been altered.

**British Library Cataloguing-in-Publication Data.
A catalogue record for this book is available from
the British Library.**

ISBN 1 874640 17 3

Typeset & Printed by
Cordfall Ltd.
0141 332 4640

To Sylvia Wachuku-King,
my guide, my boss, my friend

Contents

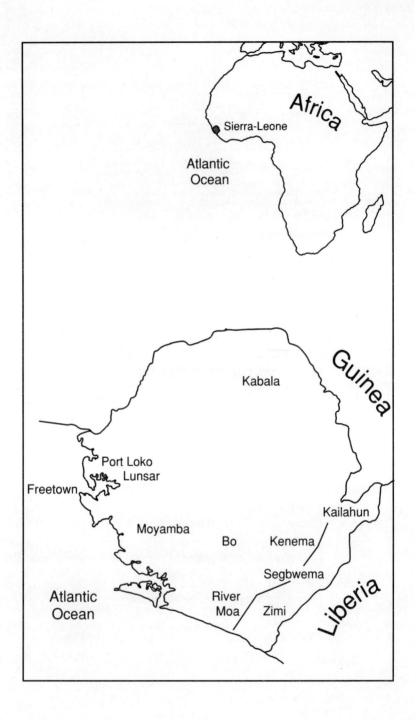

Africa

Sierra-Leone

Atlantic
Ocean

Guinea

Kabala

Port Loko
Lunsar

Freetown

Kailahun

Moyamba

Bo   Kenema

Segbwema

Atlantic
Ocean

River
Moa   Zimi

Liberia

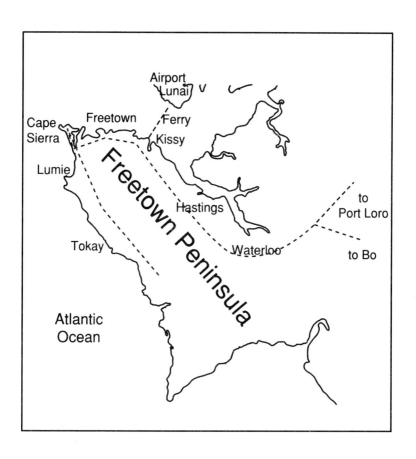

Illustrations

Acknowledgements

This book was conceived in West Africa but like the embryo kangaroo, it remained dormant and only began to grow, largely concealed from friends and family, when the environment was propitious. Even so it had a long gestation period during which some excellent ante-natal care was administered by Ann and Alan Smith, friends from my time in Sierra-Leone. Its final delivery into the world was relatively painless due to the obstetric skills of Pat Graham, whose practical help and expert advice not only corrected the errors but printed the whole manuscript so that all I had to do was cut the umbilical cord and send it out into the world.

Libby Wilson
September, 1995

Foreword

She was 64. She was due to retire from a lifetime in the National Health Service in just a year's time. The ideal moment, you might suppose, to reflect on decades of service to family planning in Britain, to put the feet up a bit, and to embrace a more self indulgent lifestyle. Instead, Dr Libby Wilson wound up in accommodation with nothing much resembling mod-cons in Sierra-Leone having responded to a request from Marie-Stopes International to lend her skills and expertise to Africa.

Her account of that sojourn is both vivid and amusing and testimony to the indefatigability of a woman who is the best kind of advertisement of what the National Health Service at least used to be about.

Ruth Wishart.
November 1994

Chapter 1 – August

Two Cold Star Beers, Now . . .

THE PLANE TOUCHED DOWN IN THE darkness of an African night. As it came to a halt I undid my safety belt and stiffly got to my feet. Sylvia was reaching up for her broad-brimmed pink straw hat, carefully stashed in the overhead locker alongside her sister's yellow one. We shuffled forward as the aircraft emptied. As I stood at the top of the mobile steps I felt the hot dampness of tropical Africa wrap round me like a wet towel. The walk across the tarmac seemed long and the surface far from smooth. The terminal buildings were dimly lit but once inside I was engulfed by a sea of noise and people. Sylvia moved confidently forward, threading her way through the conflicting aggregates of passengers and locals pressing round the various official check-points for passports, immigration, currency, health and eventually customs.

Once in the main concourse at Lungi airport bedlam took over, there appeared to be a thousand arms trying to relieve me of my hand-luggage and there were certainly at least four who got a hand on my two extremely heavy suit cases. I kept close to Sylvia and her sister who remained unperturbed by the grabbing and jostling as we squeezed our way outside to where we hoped to find the Marie-Stopes Land-Rover. They were not surprised to find that it was not there.

We made an enclave with our heavy luggage and recompensed our genuine porters appropriately, not without a noisy dispute from several blatantly false claimants, and waited in the semi-darkness.

They discussed the possible reasons for the delay in our pick-up. The ferry across the estuary was notoriously unreliable, the engine had failed more than once and recently the ship had been carried out to sea helplessly rotating, before it was eventually towed back to port. The airport generators had sufficient power to light the inside of the terminal and the only other illumination came from the headlights of the vehicles waiting to collect people.

After half an hour a battered old Land-Rover drew up and we clambered thankfully on board, the three of us squashing into the middle section as the front passenger seat was firmly occupied by a very respectably attired intelligent-looking African who supervised the proceedings. When I knew him better I came to realise that appearances can be deceptive but as he was only introduced as 'Mr Eliot' I mentally allocated to him a higher status than he either held or warranted. However, he was quite able to organise our transport to the city.

Their late arrival had been due to a delay of nearly two hours in the departure of the ferry from Freetown. This was said to be because the President had required it earlier in the day for some purpose of his own. This was reassuring in a way because at least it meant the boat was running and had not broken down.

We trundled off along the dirt road, it was dark but the faint moonlight enabled me to see that there were occasional small single story houses amid the surrounding scrub and taller trees. It seemed a long time before we reached the ferry terminal, joining a long queue that snaked away ahead of us in the gloom. Here there were more buildings and many people, walking about or grouped round tiny pinpoints of light from wicks floating in palm oil. The mosquitoes were rampant and I was glad I had remembered to pack my insect repellent in my hand-luggage. As I sat beside the open window I became aware of what appeared to be a table-top covered in little grey packets moving along just below my elbow. Sylvia leant across and said something I did not follow, whereupon the table moved out from the side of the vehicle revealing a boy of about nine carrying a tray on his head full of the local version of a 'carry-out'. I had plenty of time to realise that he was only one of many making the most of our enforced immobility and undoubted hunger, to help fill his own family's bellies on the morrow.

We were tired, having had to check-in at Heathrow at 7.30 that morning for the flight to Amsterdam where we had had quite a long wait before boarding the KLM flight to Freetown. It was now 10 o'clock and our last proper meal had been lunch in the mid-afternoon with a light snack about two hours before we landed. As we waited in the humid darkness with no sign of any movement ahead Sylvia and Mary reminisced about previous occasions when they had been stuck in the ferry queue all night.

As the queue started to move slowly forward, I could faintly see a low building ahead but no water was visible, let alone a vessel. After a further twenty minutes we had advanced two or three hundred yards and I realised that the flat blackness on my side of the Land-Rover was not land but sea, and ahead lay the ferry. The ramp into the cavernous hold was extremely steep and very narrow and I watched with horrid fascination as the KLM coach inched down the slope, its sides appearing to overhang the slipway. Our driver was obviously well-used to the exercise and we were soon packed into the darkness between a rusting truck and a state-of-the-art air-conditioned four wheel drive station wagon.

It contained an American family that had attracted my notice in the departure lounge in Amsterdam. There was Daddy, earnest, short back and sides, lightweight grey suit; Mommy, very neat, with a very large hold-all which appeared to be exactly that, as she produced out of it whatever was required for that particular situation at that particular moment; the two girls aged about fourteen and nine were similarly dressed in floral shirt waisters with little peter-pan collars and Junior, aged twelve was the epitome of clean-living healthy American boyhood with his crew cut, checked shirt with the sleeves neatly rolled up and, of course, blue jeans. I had been able to observe them for nearly an hour in the airport and was struck by their quiet behaviour, their good manners and their absence of laughter or even unrestrained smiles. They were like a family from a pre-war movie of Pollyanna. Now, here they were, returning to their mission to the heathen with all the comforts that their home base in the Mid-West could provide. The side of their luxury vehicle had the logo of an evangelical sect on its door and I have no doubt they were all totally convinced that they were doing God's will in the way He meant them to do it.

We squeezed ourselves out of the Land-Rover and just managed to find a tortuous passage between the vehicles in the noisy dark, our nostrils inhaling the fumes of petrol and diesel, clouds of which were illuminated by the headlights of the cars and trucks that were still being loaded. Eventually we found ourselves on deck and were thankful to find a bench half-way down the vessel and far enough from the latrines to enable one to breath through one's nose without nausea. Leaving Sylvia to keep my seat I leaned over the rail and looked across the oily blackness to a few faint lights on the far side of the estuary. This was my first sight of Freetown where I was going to live and work for most of the next twelve months. I thought back to how this journey had begun in Glasgow, six months before.

I was in my office in the Family Planning Centre and had just finished a half hour consultation with a couple who had great difficulty in consummating their marriage. She was an immaculate touched-up blonde, obsessional and selfish who thought sex was dirty even if its nastiness was contained in a condom and who could not allow herself to be violated. He was an intelligent, gentle man who had great difficulty in ejaculating at all and whom, I was beginning to think, was probably a repressed homosexual. I felt I had earned a cup of coffee and was reaching for the kettle when the phone rang.

"I'm Lizzie Smith from Marie-Stopes International. Your name was given to me by 'Doctors and Over-population'."

"Good Heavens, I didn't know they were still in existence. They rather lost their way after their founder, George Morris died."

"I don't really know much about them but do you remember filling in a form two or three years ago asking whether, when you retired, you would be interested in working in family planning in the Third World?"

"Yes, I do remember that, it was not so much a commitment but an indication of interest."

"Well, are you still interested? We desperately need a doctor in Sierra-Leone. . . "

That was how it had started. Naturally I had asked for a few days to think it over but in reality I think I had made my mind up within two minutes. I was nearly sixty four and would have to retire from the NHS when I reached sixty five. I had just emerged, semi-victorious, after a series of battles with the management of the Greater Glasgow Health Board. Changes in attitudes to health care and the submission of the needs of patients to the overriding gods of publicity and financial saving make it difficult for some one of my generation, whose entire professional life had been in the old style NHS, to work with the often ill-informed managerial puppets who jumped to the whims of their lay superiors. I did consider carefully whether I could usefully do much more if I stayed and decided that new ideas and ways of doing things required a fresh and younger Co-ordinator who could work with the new wave and not confront it.

I felt this opportunity was a challenge that I was fortunate to have been offered. I was fit and fairly energetic, even if overweight, I had always wanted to so some work overseas and now I would be able to, although I was a little concerned at my lack of suitable qualifications.

Marie-Stopes International was primarily a family planning organisation and I was confident that I was a genuine expert in that field. I knew from previous visits to clinics in developing countries that women were the same all over the world and my long experience working with deprived families in Glasgow had made me very aware of the fears and problems that women on low incomes have to face. I had been told that Marie-Stopes Sierra-Leone ran poly-clinics which provided general medical care because of the paucity of affordable services for the majority of the population but at that time I did not fully realise the implications.

By a fortunate coincidence Sylvia Wachuku-King, the Director of Marie-Stopes Sierra-Leone, was attending a management course in London and was due to return to Freetown at the end of July so that I would be able to travel with her. Now she was nearly home and my adventure was just beginning.

The ferry took about half an hour to cross and as we neared the land I was surprised to see that there was no urban glow over Freetown. The ferry slipway was illuminated and one or two buildings in the vicinity but the surrounding hinterland was as dark as it had been on the other side of the estuary. We clambered down the steep stairs into the hold and managed to reboard the vehicle. The next twenty minutes were like a glimpse into Hell. The ramp on this side was even steeper and just as narrow and few were rash enough to attempt to back up. Consequently every driver revved his engine, blasted his horn and tried to turn in the extremely confined space within the hold. We closed the windows as tightly as possible against the bedlam of noise and fumes but it was a useless exercise as the old Land-Rover had long ago lost the rubber seals round the windows, the doors only shut with a slam and there were numerous unintended ventilation holes in the floor and bodywork. Eventually it was our turn to manoeuvre our way up the slipway and we emerged thankfully into the open air.

We lurched up a winding pot-holed road onto a wider thoroughfare with a better surface but this respite was brief. Sylvia, Mary and I, all fairly broad in the beam, were wedged into the middle section of the Land-Rover which meant that we were thrown about much less than if we had been slimmer. The red earth of the road was scooped out into great puddles and lakes of unknowable depths with small islands of the original tarmac emerging unpredictably like volcanic atolls above the surrounding mud.

It was now after 11 o'clock and yet the streets were full of people. Along the sides of the road and spilling out into every adjacent space between the buildings and shacks which lined the street were hundreds of tiny flickering yellow lights, each dimly illuminating a metre of the surrounding darkness enough to enable the tray of fish, fruit or cooked snacks to be seen by the passers by. Men, women and children were walking purposefully along in both directions and others stood in small knots, talking together. They took their time to climb onto the raised pavements as our vehicle squelched past. In half an hour we arrived at the headquarters of the organisation in Adelaide Street. I saw the outline of a three storey building with which I later became very familiar; steel shuttered shops below, the offices and clinic in the middle and Mary's family home on the top floor. We decanted her and Mr Eliot, and drove on through much emptier streets until eventually we arrived at the Cape Sierra Hotel at the end of a mini-peninsula which jutted out into the Atlantic. It was now after midnight and the sleepy male receptionist expressed resentful surprise when we asked if any food was available. Rather grudgingly he slowly booked me in and allowed me to leave my heavy baggage beside his desk while Sylvia and I went back to the vehicle to try and find something to eat. As always, she had an immediate practical suggestion.

"There's a little beach cafe less than half a mile from here. I'm sure it'll still be open. Go along the Lumley Beach road to The Venue," she said to the driver.

We drove along beside the sea, only tussocky grass and a few tall palms between the tarmac and the sand edging the gentle ripples of the ocean. The cafe was made of palm matting over a rough hewn wooden frame. We sat at a wooden table and an audio-tape thumped out a popular Western tune with a strong rhythm but it was not too loud or intrusive. We were the only people there.

"What would you like?" asked Sylvia.

"I've almost got past being hungry – I couldn't eat much but I'm terribly thirsty," I replied. "I quite fancy something hot and savoury, I don't mean peppery hot, just hot hot!"

"I know the very thing, a shawama, its a savoury Lebanese pancake, but first things first." She looked up at the smiling waiter, standing expectantly beside us.

"Two cold Star beers NOW and two shawamas to follow."

So it was that the first drink I had in Sierra-Leone was its very own Star which established a precedent which I followed whenever I could for the rest of my stay and the first food was Lebanese which introduced me to the all pervading and long established influence of these Middle-Eastern gentlemen in West Africa.

Sylvia had insisted that I had a sea view and I certainly had a most beautiful site for my room. It was at the end of a long arm consisting of three horizontal two-storey blocks. I was on the first floor and looked straight out over the ocean with only thirty yards of scrubby grass and two or three palm trees between me and the beach. One great advantage, in addition to the view, was that it was nearly always windy and during the day or when the air-conditioning was not working at night I could open the window and enjoy a refreshing breeze off the sea.

I was picked up next morning by Sylvia in the Marie-Stopes Peugeot. This vehicle was in a very precarious state and was due to be replaced but on this occasion it crawled along provided we stopped every two miles to fill it up with water. I was taken to the main clinic at Collegiate School Road where I met the staff. Then we went on to Adelaide Street to meet the people in the office and the nurses who ran the small clinic there. Everyone was very friendly and cheerful and I was made to feel genuinely welcome.

I negotiated with a taxi driver from the hotel pool to take me into the Post Office in the centre of the town and to pick me up there an hour later, for what I knew was the outrageous sum of 1600 leones. I had no real alternative and I had not yet developed the bargaining skills I acquired later. The Post Office is a grim concrete building but cool inside. This was the only place at which one could post mail as it contained the only letterbox in Freetown. I learnt later that in theory there were other boxes but as they never appeared to be emptied they were not used. It was also the only place where one could buy stamps and, at that time, was where I had to go to collect my mail.

I posted two letters and then walked round the centre of the town. I had never seen anywhere that was so run down and decrepit. The differences between the buildings was very noticeable – there were a few modern constructions several stories high, in particular that of the Standard Chartered Bank of America which also contained the British High Commission. This was the tallest block in Freetown. It was almost unique in having lifts which did work at times. Some of the other government buildings were also quite large although the Treasury looked as though it had not had a coat of paint since it was built, probably in the last century. Every time I passed it had shed a few more fragments of stone or plaster onto the rubble on the side-walk. In between were two and three-storey colonial buildings which must once have been very elegant but now the balconies were falling to bits, the clap-boarding coming off and the tin roofs patched or even with visible holes. In the gaps between there were groups of little shacks of corrugated iron nailed onto some kind of wooden frame, not even whole sheets of corrugated iron but

23

patchworks of different sizes and shapes with stones on the roofs to prevent them flying off in a storm. They were built straight onto the earth which, in the rainy season as it was then, meant liquid mud.

I bought a second-hand children's atlas because it contained a map of Freetown and also of Sierra-Leone. In it were maps showing the seasonal temperatures and relative humidity and I was interested to see that there was remarkably little variation throughout the year although, naturally there were big differences in rainfall.

In the afternoon I walked along the ocean-washed sands of Lumley beach, which stretches from the hotel for nearly two miles as far as the distant point. I wandered along below the high-water mark carrying my camera, binoculars and bird book in a small rucksack, hoping to find exotic shells or mysterious flotsam. Alas, it was not that kind of beach and if anything interesting was washed up I am sure one of the raggle taggle mob of beach boys would have found it first. I set myself a target to reach and then returned; on the walk I was approached several times by men trying to sell me things but they were not aggressive and I never felt threatened. I found out subsequently that it was considered unwise to go further than about half a mile from the hotel as there had been muggings and bag-snatchings. I'm glad I did not know this at the time because I thoroughly enjoyed my stroll and my first paddle in the Atlantic in West Africa.

On Sunday Sylvia and her three children came to visit me in the afternoon. It was good to meet her family even if they were a little over-awed at first. I was amazed to find out that because she lives some way up the hill in Lumley, which makes it more pleasant, the water pressure is so low that they had had no running water for four months; every drop had to be carried in drums from a friend's house lower down the hill. The children carry these drums on their heads, even the nine year old managed a five gallon drum uphill for more than half a mile.

Monday was my first working day at a clinic. It was in a single storey bungalow which had formerly been a private house. It was too small and had been badly converted for its present purpose. There was no system of 'flow' for the clients and consequently people were constantly squeezing past one another and waiting in narrow passages with the minimum of privacy for consultations and nursing procedures. In spite of these difficulties an average of fifty patients were seen every day and, on ante-natal days, many more, the staff remaining cheerful and friendly throughout.

On this Monday another doctor and myself, Sister Cline, Sister Meux, Lauretta, Mamie and Admiah the girl in the caged-in sentry box known as the dispensary, attended to the needs of fifty-nine people. The other doctor was a Russian who had met her husband in Moscow where he was also a medical student in the post-colonial era when newly independent Sierra-Leone had been courted by the USSR. In addition to the female staff there was a young man who was supposed to clear the encroaching grass and undergrowth, look after the generator, fetch water from the outside tap (I soon discovered that although there was a basin in the consulting room nothing happened when I turned on the tap), and wash the floors inside the building once the clients had gone. There was also a night watchman who had only recently been appointed as his predecessor had been suspected of being implicated in the theft of the previous generator.

Most of the patients were medical cases, many of them children and only three or four wanted family planning. Later in the morning I watched the Russian doctor do four menstrual extractions, the local euphemism for abortions. I found this distressing on a number of counts. The women were placed in the lithotomy position on a couch, ie they were semi reclining with their legs supported by stirrups, their thighs wide apart. Then, without any anaesthetic, a suction curette with a large syringe attached to a plastic cannula was inserted through the opening in the cervix, or neck of the uterus. Precautions against cross infection were extremely poor, the same syringe was used several times with only the cannula being changed. The first woman screamed and moaned and the Doctor said sharply, "Stop it."

Turning to me she said, "These women can have six or seven children with no problems. This is a painless procedure, she is just making a fuss."

The nurse, trained by this doctor, was present solely to make sure the instruments were available, and did nothing to comfort the patient or hold her hand. I asked whether there was ever anybody to talk the woman through the procedure but was told that this was totally unnecessary and would be "just pampering to them".

The two succeeding operations were not quite so unpleasant but the last one was a woman who was almost certainly more than twelve weeks pregnant and she also found the operation extremely painful and upsetting; the syringe sucked out quantities of blood, well over half a pint as well as the bulky products of conception. There was too much blood to be contained in the kidney dish and it spilt everywhere making the scene of the operation resemble an old-fashioned butcher's shop. The spillage and splashes were mopped up with the same towel that was used for every patient but as that was the last case for the morning at least no other poor frightened woman was exposed to the evidence of what her predecessors had been through.

Treatment prescribed for the medical cases was of the poly-pharmacy variety, at least two antibiotics, panadol (paracetamol), phenergan (an anti-histamine with noticeable sedative side effects), and always quantities of vitamins, especially B Co (vitamin B compound) preferably by injection. Scabies was treated not only with the local application of benzoyl-benzoate lotion but also with phenergan. Children with coughs were given phenergan 'three times a day', presumably to keep them asleep all the time. All children who were old enough not to be fully breast fed were regarded, probably correctly, as having worms and were automatically given anti-worm treatment, those running a fever which was not obviously due to a chest infection were treated for malaria. As the majority of the patients were diagnosed and treated by the nursing staff this blanket type medication was probably justified and was unlikely to do harm, but problems arose when the client could only afford a few of the products on the prescription and was likely to choose the cheapest, eg the vitamins, and not buy the essential ampicillin for her toddler with pneumonia.

Later I went with Sylvia to the Department of Immigration as I had only a three month visa and I would need a resident's permit. We were told there would be no problem about this as long as I had a letter from the Department of Health stating that I was working as a doctor for a year with the Marie-Stopes Society. I was unaware then that my permit would eventually reach me six weeks after I arrived back in Scotland the following summer!

After these necessary chores were completed we went from the centre of the town through the slums of Kissy to Wellington. The crowded streets, the dirt and the poverty made the British names on the streets and miserable back alleys seem like an ironic comment; Bathhurst Street, Circular Road, Goderich Street, and even Elba Street, a reminder, like Wellington and Waterloo, of the time when the colony was founded. Virtually all the women, most of the children, and some of the men carried burdens on their heads, rarely supported by a hand. One man was carrying a calor gas cylinder, another an obviously full bucket, the women carried basins of wet washing, trays, usually made of woven cane or fibre and often bearing whatever items they were trying to sell.

On the following Saturday Sylvia picked me up in the Land-Rover just after nine and took me to Wilkinson Road as the Collegiate School Road clinic was often perversely referred to. Saturdays were rarely busy and the heavy rain also contributed to the paucity of clients. This was a bonus as far as I was concerned as it gave me more time with each patient and enabled me to talk to the nurses without the pressure of knowing there was a waiting room full of patients. I was explaining to a woman about a coil (a type of intra-uterine contraceptive device) when Sister came in and asked me to see a very small baby who was seriously ill. The child was forty eight hours old and had been delivered at home by a traditional birth attendant (TBA) and was having tetanic spasms. She was probably going to die and all I could do was to give the aunt who had brought her to the clinic a note to the Children's Hospital and tell her to take the child there as soon as possible. This was the second neonate I had seen in two days.

The day before a little girl of seven days old had been brought in with a grossly distended abdomen, a tiny emaciated thing whose mother was still in hospital with eclampsia (high blood pressure associated with pregnancy and child-birth). She obviously had an obstruction, whether this was due to some congenital abnormality or to an intususseption (impacted kinking of the bowel) I was not skilled enough to tell, but immediate surgery was the only thing that would give her a chance of life. The sensible and concerned grandmother took the baby to hospital straight away and fortunately had the means to cover the cost of the operation. Unlike general practitioners in the UK we never had any communication from hospital staff about the outcome of such referrals, but five months later a young mother brought in a lively attractive and well nourished baby girl beautifully dressed in a pretty pink frock with matching bootees. The child had a trivial rash but the real reason for the visit was to thank us for, as she believed, saving her daughter's life. We probably did, as surgical intervention delayed for a further two or three hours would have almost certainly been too late.

The next patient was Helmut, a very different child from the miserable eight year old who had come in the day before. His mother had cut his arm quite badly with a knife when she struck him because he had damaged a plastic bucket. He was a Liberian refugee but the mother and three children were staying with a local family. He was terrified and screamed and screamed but it was essential that we put two stitches into the cut on his arm. It was with very great difficulty that this was attempted. He moved the first time so that the needle broke in the wound.

27

This resulted in even more trauma extracting it and then a bigger needle had to be used to complete the job. When it was done he was rewarded, at his own request, with a present of empty syringe, minus the needle, of course. Then, when he had had his anti-tetanus injection, during which he again raised the roof, he was given that syringe as well, whereupon his tears dried up rapidly. On this morning he marched in all smiles, very proud of the bandage on his arm and friends with every one. He could speak quite good English as did most of the Liberians, whereas few Sierra-Leonians of primary school age could speak it at all. Helmut had a most attractive smile and I was sure he would come back on Monday to have the wound looked at. I was afraid it would probably become infected, as indeed it did, but even so it healed quite quickly.

After him there were the usual cases of diarrhoea and vomiting, coughs and fevers and a little French boy of two brought by his African nanny. He had some infected bites on his arm. He usually attended a private doctor but she was out of town that weekend so the nurse maid had brought him to see us. The treatment was simple, he only needed some fucidin ointment and fortunately we had this in the dispensary. He was not ill but the lesions looked rather unpleasant. He whined nearly all the time asking for a "biccy". This was in marked contrast to the African children who are long-suffering and undemanding. He was the only whining child I ever encountered in a Marie-Stopes clinic.

One evening in late August I was finishing my meal in the dining room of the Cape Sierra. It had not been a very exciting gastronomic experience but it was adequate even if all too familiar. I had been reading a book throughout the meal, the latest Ruth Rendell, brought with me from home and saved for these first weeks in Sierra-Leone. I usually sat at one particular table because it combined a strategic position vis-à-vis the waiter, who was liable to overlook diners who were in corners far from the servery, and was well lit, being directly under one of the few overhead lights. I finished a chapter and, raising my head looked properly round the room. I was surprised to see another white-haired lady in late middle-age sitting near the door, also reading a book while she ate. As I made my way out I could see she was deep in *The Silence of the Lambs*. A potential kindred spirit; I stopped and introduced myself. This was the beginning of a happy and continuing friendship which was a great support to me, and, I believe, to her, in the following months.

Leona, like me, was staying in the Cape Sierra while she sought for more permanent accommodation. She had been sent to Freetown to be the new director of a large Catholic Aid agency. She said nothing about the reasons for her sudden translation to Africa and naturally I did not ask but snippets of golf-club gossip crossed my mind. I remembered hearing of a major scandal involving the rapid departure of the previous director, a black American priest, and the sacking of eight or nine of the top management because of involvement in serious corruption. Leona had been sent to clean up the mess with hardly any of the original staff and no knowledge of Africa. She had worked previously for the same agency in Thailand, Jordan and Jerusalem but was, in fact, a nun, seconded from her order to work wherever in the world there were refugees and poverty. Sierra-Leone, being the poorest country in the world had been a needy recipient of the agency's help when the civil war in Liberia, with which it has a common boundary, plunged the agency into the thick of the refugee crisis.

We arranged to go out together the following evening for a meal at one of the beach-side restaurants along the Lumley peninsula, a pleasure I had not been able to enjoy so far, on my own, and without transport. This was the first of an almost weekly rendezvous. By the end of August Leona had installed herself in a self-catering flat in another nearby hotel, the Bintumani. As she lent it to me whenever she was away for more than forty-eight hours I became very familiar with it but in those early weeks the bonus I relished most when I visited her was the superb view from her little balcony, drinking in the sunsets over the Atlantic as we enjoyed our Star beer. Then, off to 'George's' or 'Grass Roots' in her agency Peugeot for a pleasant seafood meal under the palms with the sea lapping gently on the sand. We always had plenty to talk about and if work was mentioned it concerned the practical problems of coping with everyday life and not personalities or office gossip. It was remarkable to me to find that I had so many common interests with, and similar views to, an American Roman Catholic nun. We enjoyed the same books, neither having the mental stamina to read anything heavier than Dickens and both finding a good detective story almost as relaxing as a gin and tonic and certainly with a longer lasting effect.

My own attempts to find accommodation were less happy. Marie-Stopes is a small charity and the principle governing their Aid programmes was that each should be self-financing within a given period of time. The employment of a European doctor was obviously an expensive item although I was only paid the equivalent of £200 a month in local money. I bought a car myself and paid for it in sterling through my UK bank and Marie-Stopes paid for the fuel (but not the punctures).

I sold the Fiesta to Marie-Stopes Sierra-Leone at its UK valuation when I returned home, which proved a satisfactory arrangement to both parties. My living quarters were to be their responsibility and the cost of any type of hotel flat was away beyond their means. The hotels were swarming with wealthy Liberian refugees who had managed to escape from Monrovia with their chauffeur driven Mercedes and Peugeots, their stewards and nannies. Although I was not competing for their brand of rented accommodation there were many other less opulent, but far from bankrupt, displaced persons who wanted much the same sort of home as I did. At that time I did not have the contacts with expatriates who might have been able to help. I had not appreciated, at first, that it was essential to be housed in a secure compound with watchmen, especially at night, not only for my own protection but because of the car.

Towards the end of the month Sylvia said she had found a possible flat. I suspect she had known about it all along but had waited to see if anything better turned up.

"It's in a bungalow belonging to a Mr Brown – that's what he calls himself because he's Indian and no one can say his proper name. He lives in the main part with his wife and family," she explained.

"They had a single professional lady living in it for a year but its been empty for months now because Mrs Brown doesn't want a single man or a family living underneath her."

The bungalow was in Wilkinson Road, about a mile from the main clinic. It was bounded on the front and right-hand side by a high wall of concrete topped with broken glass and on the left by a tall fence and thick thorn hedge separating it from the next house. The entrance gates were shut and we drew off the road onto the wide verge in front of the adjacent Kingdom Hall, a centre for the Seventh Day Adventists. We scrambled out of the Land-Rover and Sylvia peered through a crack in the solid wooden gates. She rattled them energetically and told our driver to hoot the horn. After several minutes an old man shuffled slowly across the compound and undid the cross-bar. We walked over to the front door and tried ringing the bell but as there was no power we resorted to a gentle knock. When this failed to produce a response, Musu, as I subsequently learnt was the old man's name, called out, "Missus, Missus," and the door was unlocked from the inside.

Mrs Brown was a plump comfortable Indian lady who invited us into her living room and offered us tea. The room was dark and was heavily furnished with upholstered settees and armchairs round the sides which left a small rectangular space in the middle.

Sylvia introduced me and said I would be working for Marie-Stopes for the next year and wanted accommodation for myself and my car.

"We let the flat to a very nice single Indian lady for two years but then her work contract was up and she had to go home. I do not want a family with children in it, I've plenty of my own with my grandchildren as well."

She led the way out of her front door and down the side of the bungalow which was built on a considerable slope. The concrete path was broken and uneven and a continuous stream of water fanned out over the rough surface so that one's feet were inevitably wet by the time the flat terrace at the back was reached.

"There is small problem with pipe, it will be fixed by the week-end," she explained. The back of the building was faced with a concrete wall up to the height of the first floor, solid for the lower four feet and the upper part latticed by a regular pattern of fenestrations. Inside this wall there was a corridor shaped space, four feet wide bounded on the inside by the back of the original building. The outer door was open but the inner was closed with a large padlock which she undid and ushered us inside. We were in a spacious 'hall', half divided by a central support, with two doors opening off each side. There was an overwhelming atmosphere of gloom and damp which was off-putting at first. The windows opened into the dead space behind the protecting wall and little light percolated through to the rooms behind. The outer wall of the room to the left lay along the course of the permanent spring outside and it was obvious that "small problem with pipe" had been present for months and probably longer. The plaster was sodden and an old bedstead and mattress were disintegrating with rust and mould; no wonder the place smelt of damp. However, the room on the opposite side looked quite promising, it was dry and had a window in the side wall that opened directly onto the path round the house between the thorn hedge and the bungalow. The kitchen was also on this side and was light and caught any little breeze that might be blowing. The other unexpected bonus was that although the shower, washbasin and separate lavatory were on the damp side of the flat, there was an excellent supply of clean drinkable water which came straight from the mains water pipe. The high pressure was due to Wilkinson Road being at sea level. The disadvantage of the location was that over the high wall at the back of the garden were mangrove swamps, the ideal breeding ground for mosquitoes.

"I think I could manage here," I said. "I could use this room as a bed-sit and provided I have an air-conditioner and a fridge I'll be fine."

"What about the power?" said Sylvia to Mrs Brown.

"No problem, my husband has paid large dash to Power Company so that we are on same supply as lady-friend of the President. Of course, nobody has power during day except at weekends but we have it nearly every night until next morning."

I was relieved to hear this as I knew from comments of the nurses that the supply to most parts of Freetown was infrequent and erratic.

Sylvia and I parted from Mrs Brown, telling her we would think it over and let her husband know before the end of the week. I knew that this was the only practical solution for the time being although it had many drawbacks. If I had known then that the President's wife, who had been abroad for four years, would return within six weeks of my taking up residence and that, whether as a consequence or not, the power would be almost totally discontinued, perhaps I would not have agreed so readily.

Once the decision was made Sylvia lost no time in getting the flat cleaned, a fresh coat of paint on the walls and installing a large fridge and an air-conditioner and within a week I had moved in. The bed was slightly wider than the standard British 3ft 6 but this marginally increased comfort was more than mitigated by the mattress which was technically 'interior sprung'. The springs had ceased springing many tropical moons before and three had uncoiled their way through the nearly rotten ticking and were lying in wait for my unsuspecting flesh concealed by the mattress cover. I spent the first night in some discomfort, trying to lie on my side without impaling myself on the three projecting wires. The next day, in daylight, I managed to cut off about half an inch of each offending spring with the pliers I had brought with me, but I knew this treatment was only palliative and the problem would recur.

Amongst my excess baggage was a thick cardboard tryptich displaying the male and female reproductive cycles in great detail. I decided that this could be sacrificed in order to ensure me a reasonable nights sleep and trisected it accordingly. I introduced the panels through a pre-existing lateral slit in the cover and slid them over each offending spike. This was effective and it was easy to adjust their positions if they became displaced. Two pillows were bought at Choitrams, the 'super-market' in the centre of the town; they were fat and bulgy and filled with little cubes of foam plastic which had a very characteristic smell and made them very inflexible but they were adequate for their purpose.

I had brought a mosquito net with me but when I examined it I realised that it was made to be suspended from a hook in the ceiling and as there was no hook I could not use it. This meant that all the windows had to be firmly closed, before dusk if possible and I regularly sprayed my living room with 'Killit' or whatever anti-insect spray I could get hold of. I did mention the problem to Sylvia but she was so busy and had so many other more pressing matters to deal with, that I felt I could not go on nagging about it.

Many months later I decided I must get it fixed, partly because of the horror of my friends when they found out I had no net and my flat was immediately beside the mangrove swamps. Eventually a blacksmith was found who welded a huge hook onto an iron plate. This was in turn fixed to a flat wooden base which could be nailed to the ceiling over my bed. No attempt was made to find out where the underlying wooden beams lay under the plaster and sometimes when I had inadvertently wrenched the net as I tried to tuck it in, I wondered if the risk of being knocked out, or worse by a large iron structure descending on my head from a height was not greater than contracting malaria. It was certainly much more complicated to go to bed once I had the net. The mattress was about four inches too wide to fit properly inside, consequently I could tuck in three sides but I had to leave the fourth open until I had crawled in myself. Then the difficulties began as it is very awkward to tuck something under the mattress one is lying on, particularly when there is insufficient material and it does not stretch. It was only possible by bending up the sides of the mattress so that it became a bit like a rubber dinghy. All this had usually to be done in darkness and entailed very careful planning to make sure there was nothing I could possibly want before I retreated into my cocoon for the night.

Mrs Brown also arranged for me to have the services of James to do my laundry and clean the flat. He was sixteen years old and had lost his parents 'up-country' but his grandmother lived in Freetown. He spoke good English and had been at school until he was thirteen, he told me later. I asked how much I should pay him as he was already employed by my landlady for several hours each day.

"Oh, you don't want to give him too much, he gets a good meal here every day as well as his wages."

"Do you mean about 1,000 leones?" This was equivalent to £3 at the current rate of exchange.

"Well, Doctor Wilson, that would do every two months but you should only pay him once a week, a hundred and fifty at the most."

I made no further comment but paid the boy three hundred regularly and more if he did the ironing. I soon found out that 'James' was not his real name as Mrs Brown had 'christened' him this when he had entered her employment. His 'room' was one end of the space between the outer and inner walls of my flat, about four feet across and six long. He had no privacy and each time I let myself in after an evening with Leona or at the golf club I was aware that this other human being was sleeping on a piece of cardboard on the cement floor with his only possession, another shirt, hanging over a wire stretched as a clothes line above his head. After a week or two he asked me to look after his pathetically small savings as he was afraid the night watchmen might steal from him. He was saving up to buy a pair of trainers which, at the amounts he could save, was going to take many years.

I had brought a small travelling iron out with me and in those early weeks, still had power for a few hours at weekends. I gave James the iron and plugged it in for him showing him how to adjust the heat. I gave him my best pair of jeans and left him in the kitchen to get on with it. I was half way through a letter to one of my daughters when I became aware of a significant signal to my nose. Poor James and poor jeans. He had never used an electric iron before but had not liked to lose face by admitting it. When he realised that I was not going to be cross with him he was amazed; I gathered that the usual reaction to a singed garment would have been a beating. He suggested asking Mrs Brown if he could borrow the flat-iron from upstairs which was heated directly on the stove. She was agreeable and after that there were no disasters with my laundry. He was very skilled with the primitive iron, much as my grandmother must have been. I came to like James a lot and am sure that he was honest but our association was not to last for long.

One evening six weeks after I took up residence in Wilkinson Road, I returned home to hear his voice raised in heartrending distress within his concrete walls. He was not aware of my approach and I could hear him praying aloud, "Oh my Lord Jesus Christ I have tried to do your will. I tell the truth, help me, help me I pray you. . . " He was sobbing and I knew he would not want his anguish to be witnessed by another, however sympathetic. I retreated silently and then walked noisily down the slope beside the house shouting "Goodbye" to a non-existent friend, before crunching loudly over the gritty concrete as I approached my door. He heard me and fell silent. I let myself into the passageway, using my torch to unlock the padlock on the inner door and said, Goodnight, James in my usual fashion. The next morning he told me he had been told to leave that day.

"But why? What have you done?"

34

"Mrs Brown say I use scissors to try and break into car to steal cassette player."

"But you haven't got any scissors!"

"I borrow scissors from Mrs Brown to cut my hair. I forgot to give them back straight away. Mr Brown says he find scratch marks round keyhole on his car so I must go. No reference."

"Where will you go?" I asked him. "What will you do?"

"I go to my grandmother. Something will turn up." He grinned, a most engaging grin, his distress of the night before put behind him, at least for the present.

"I believe you didn't do it. It would have been such a stupid thing to do. You would be the first suspect and I know you are not stupid and I believe you are honest." I shook hands with him and pressed 1000 leones into his hand.

"This is to help your grandmother feed you until you can get another job, and here is your envelope with your savings. The very best of luck, James." I felt guilty as I said this because I had never mastered the pronunciation of his true name and felt that in not taking enough trouble to do so, I was almost on a par with Mrs Brown.

Months later I was stuck in a traffic jam in Congo Road when I heard a happy shout from a vehicle similarly halted, going in the opposite direction.

"Doctah Wilson, Doctah Wilson, it's me, James." He was standing in the back of an open truck with the logo of the Aerated Water Company on the cab.

"My friend got me a job with the bottling company and now I am learning to drive. Soon I will not just be loading, I will be driver!" He looked fit and happy and had filled out since October and had become a very good looking young man. I was delighted to see him and managed to shout this across to him before the unscrambling of the traffic carried us away in opposite directions.

Chapter 2 – September

Keep Calm, Think . . .

I SAT AT THE SMALL TABLE-DESK IN THE 'consulting room' behind the blue curtain at Collegiate School Road, writing a letter while I waited to be picked up. The nurses were balancing the day's takings and completing the numerous records required by the office before the clinic could be locked up and we could all go home. The shiny back of a calendar lay under my fore-arm to prevent the thin paper of the air-letter from buckling with my sweat. Lauretta's smiling face appeared round the curtain,

"It's an emergency Doc, will you see him?"

I quickly swept my letter and other bits and pieces into the drawer and turned to welcome the mother and baby. The child was about two years old and not seriously ill. He had a rash, not the ubiquitous scabies but probable measles. He had a mild chest infection which might get worse so I prescribed ampicillin syrup and half a paediatric paracetamol every four hours. If I had not been there, the nurses would have given him at least six other medicaments which his mother could not afford. As it was, the syrup took nearly all her money. An injection of penicillin would have cost less but need to be repeated daily for three days and there was no guarantee that the woman would return. I still did not realise at that time what great emphasis Africans place on injections but I had seen a six month old baby with a huge fluctuating abscess in her thigh that morning from an intramuscular injection given, I am glad to say, at another clinic.

While I had been dealing with the patient the staff had completed their tasks and only Sister Cline was left waiting to lock up. The old Land-Rover had arrived and we gave her a lift home. She lived nearby, down a rough lane, off the main road. She had had a busy day, we were late and she was returning to cook her own and her husband's main meal on a charcoal fire outside the back door of her comfortable modern house, because there was no power.

My feelings about these delays were mixed as I was being taken to the British High Commission compound to pick up the car I had bought from one of their staff who was returning to London. I was very excited at the thought of being able to go where and when I liked, no longer having to wait, sometimes for nearly an hour, before being picked up to go to work and not having to ask almost complete strangers to give me a lift to the golf club on Thursday evenings for my weekly intake of excellent fish and chips (not to mention the games of darts).

On the other hand, I was terrified of driving on the Sierra-Leonian roads and so had planned the car collection well before dark, with an initial run along the Beach Road to the Cape-Sierra Hotel to have my hair done. I duly arrived at the British High Commission and completed the formalities. The keys were handed over and I got behind the wheel, on the left hand side of course. Sylvia had waited in the Land-Rover to escort me down the long sweep of Spur Road before being taken to her own house away up Juba Hill, while I carried on right, towards the sea and the beach.

Vivienne was a Cornish woman who had met her Sierra-Leonian husband when he was attending the Cambourne School of Mines and she was training to be a hairdresser. Their marriage had broken up many years before but Viv enjoyed her life in West Africa in spite of its drawbacks. She had many friends of many nationalities and earned enough to live on doing the hair of ex-pats like me, regular customers amongst the Lebanese, and, at that time, the non-African refugees from Liberia who were staying in the hotel where her salon was.

The timing of the appointment for a shampoo and set was crucial. The management of the Cape-Sierra did not start their generator until 6 o'clock but it was beginning to get dark by half past so it was necessary to have the rollers in place and be poised to screw oneself under the antique dryer on the dot of the hour. My hair did not take long to dry – ten minutes or so and I delved into my brief case to find the huge wad of dirty notes needed to pay. I scrabbled amongst the detritus, lifted out the thermos flask I'd used for my midday tea, the empty plastic bag that had held my unbuttered piece of bread and the single foil-wrapped segment of tasteless cheese, the British National Formulary and various notes I had made on different patients. A monstrous hand twisted my gut as I realised I had lost my wallet.

"Keep calm." I adjured myself. "Think."

I realised I must have left it at the British High Commission compound when I collected the car. Vivienne was happy to trust me – she hadn't much option, but she knew me well enough by this time. I drove back the way I had come – there was little traffic and the road surface was relatively free from pot-holes. I was not really worried but was looking forward to a blissful cold shower and a change from my sweaty clothes. Unfortunately an extensive search at the British High Commission failed to reveal the wallet. I decided that it must have fallen from my lap when I had had the lift in the Land-Rover. The only thing to do was to go back home and try and ring Sylvia on my Indian landlord's phone. As I waited for the watchman to open the seven foot gates in response to my toot, the full horror of my situation dawned on me. It was not only money that lived in my wallet, it was my keys!

My landlady was very kind and tried to make the connection for me but as was the norm in Freetown at that time, this proved to be impossible. She then offered me a cup of tea which in my state of heat, sweat, and frustration was even more welcome than a Star beer would have been.

As I cooled down and became more rational I started to think properly and retraced my movements before I reached the British High Commission the first time. I remembered suddenly sweeping my writing materials into the drawer when the baby arrived unexpectedly at the clinic, perhaps the wallet was there as well?

I knew Sister Cline had the keys to the clinic and, because we had given her a lift home, I knew, more or less, where she lived. I thanked my landlady warmly (in every sense of the word) and once more got behind the wheel, only now the tropical dusk was rapidly turning into night. Fortunately the light switches and controls on the Ford Fiesta were similar to the car I had had in the UK. I had not studied the manual, having no intention of driving in the dark until I was confident in daylight.

I set off down Wilkinson Road, back past the clinic – was Sister Cline's turning the second or third on the left? I knew it was narrow with little indication from the street.

Ah, here it was. A tight turn and, as soon as I was in it, I knew it was the wrong one. It was even rougher and so narrow I had no choice but to continue down past the curious eyes of the entire population of every shack within a hundred yards, or so it seemed to me. I was in imminent danger of slaughtering numerous bedraggled hens or even permanently injuring a goat. It was a cul-de-sac and the blind end was only a yard or two wider than the rest. After a six-point turn I started back lurching over boulders, tilting wildly first to one side then the other before descending into a miniature pond and crawling out the other side. All was well until I reached the final access onto the tarmaced main road where the dirt had crumbled away and left a sharp step of about six inches on the off-side.

Disaster struck as I tried to circumnavigate the problem. There was a horrid whistling rush of air and the tyre was as flat as a pancake. I manage to pull the car round onto the main road, got out and asked a passer-by if he knew where Sister Cline lived. It was the next turning on the left.

I struggled down the uneven track in my unsuitable shoes recollecting the landmarks as I went. Sister had changed from her smart Marie-Stopes uniform into clothes more appropriate for cooking on an open fire but she welcomed me and introduced me to her husband, an accountant with a big building firm. They immediately went into action. Sister changed into her street clothes and Mr Cline drove us both back to the main road where I was relieved to see the Fiesta had not been molested. Mr Cline took charge and he was quickly surrounded by several young men all keen to change the wheel. He was obviously in complete control of the situation and he urged his wife and me to hurry along to the clinic.

"By the time you have got there and unlocked the place and found what you are looking for and come back here, the wheel will be changed and you will be keeping me waiting," he expostulated. We hurried along the roadside in the dark, the distance seemed much further than it had in the car but it was only about a third of a mile. Once there, we had to attract the attention of the watchman to open the padlock on the gates of the compound. Protocol then demanded that the bunch of a dozen or so keys were handed to him to unlock the three separate padlocks and Yale lock on the door into the building. This was a new night watchman and he was unfamiliar with the keys but reluctant to say so. I now knew enough to keep my mouth shut and hide my impatience as best I could. At least Sister had brought a torch but even so it seemed to take old Abu a very long time before he fitted the right key into each keyhole and we were inside. There remained two more internal doors to open but Sister had no trouble in undoing them herself and I was at last able to open the drawer in my desk in the consulting room.

There was my wallet, intact, just as I had swept it out of sight four hours before. We had to reverse all the security procedures, thanked Abu for his help and hurried back to Mr Cline who, as he had promised, had supervised the changing of the wheel and was sitting in his own car keeping guard over them both. He told me I should take the punctured tyre to a nearby garage in the morning where it would be repaired for 80 leones (about 30p) but he would strongly advise getting inner tubes fitted as they could be repaired more easily and cheaply than tubeless tyres. I thanked my rescuers and drove back home with considerable trepidation as there were no street lights and cars and trucks were frequently parked on the main road and never had any lights. As I drove gingerly along I suddenly realised that it was now long after 7 o'clock and that Sylvia was going to pick me up 'soon after seven' to take me to an engagement ceremony.

I arrived at the compound gate and pressed the horn quickly three times to attract the attention of the watchmen. Fortunately it was too early for them to have fallen asleep and the bolts were withdrawn promptly and I was able to drive in. Thank goodness I did not have to drive anywhere else tonight, I had had enough trauma behind a wheel for one day. I locked the car and hurried in darkness down the concrete slope that led to the back of the building and my front door. At last I was able to get inside the flat and have a shower. I flicked on the switch, no response, then I realised the significance of the unlit compound. There was no power!

Fortunately, on this occasion anyway, Sylvia was nearly always late. It was now 7.40pm and I was so sweaty that I had great difficulty stripping off my dress but the bliss of standing under the full force of the shower washed away the stresses of the evening. I dressed with some difficulty by the light of one candle and Sylvia arrived to collect me before I was quite ready but I only kept her waiting five minutes and then sank gratefully beside her into the back of the Marie-Stopes Peugeot.

We drove through the city until we came to the turn off for Fourah Bay College or, as it is now called, The University of Sierra-Leone. The campus was on a magnificent site, high on the ridge overlooking the ocean and the buildings were scattered amongst tall mature trees. I was told that the gardens had once been beautiful but now they were largely untended and native scrub had inevitably taken over.

Esther lived with her family in a pleasant bungalow within the campus about half a mile from the main university buildings. The dirt side roads had no names but we easily found the right house because there were several vehicles parked outside and we could see in the moonlight a group of men gathered round the front door. We were a little late and had arrived at the point in the engagement ceremony when the future husband's advocate was knocking firmly on the closed door asking for admission. We waited outside, well clear of the bridegroom's entourage, while Sylvia briefed me. The man and woman who wish to be engaged each choose a spokesman to represent them and plead their case. Originally these were probably their fathers but nowadays the roles are played by semi-professional elder statesmen who know the family and are practised orators. The future husband sends a delegation led by his spokesman to the home of his intended but he himself is not present. The ritual follows a regular pattern with which everyone is familiar and, being Africa, it is somewhat lengthy. The admission ceremony lasted about a quarter of an hour and then the supplicant and his party were allowed in.

We followed closely, as inconspicuously as possible. There were about thirty people sitting round the sides of the room in half darkness leaving a clear space for the drama to be played out. This entailed very long speeches by the 'professional' advocates in rolling cadences and in words that were a mixture of the King James Bible and Anthony Trollope. There was a repeated request for a sight of the 'beautiful pink rose' which had been observed in the garden and which was the only one which could satisfy the young man's desire.

Eventually the wish appeared to be granted and one of the young female relatives went out of the room, not without many smiles and giggles, to return with a handsome young lady dressed in red. Alas, although this rose was undoubtedly lovely she was not the pink rose of his heart's delight. Three more young women were introduced unsuccessfully and when it was time for the fifth there was a considerable delay and a lot of whispering and giggling before a delightful little girl of about four years old wearing a pretty yellow dress came half shyly into the room. There were claps and shouts and a great deal of laughter before the company settled down to welcome the next candidate. This one was received even more vociferously as it proved to be a child of seven or so in a lovely green dress but who happened to be a boy!

At last it was Esther's turn, and there she was in a very attractive pink outfit looking absolutely stunning but with the same warm smile that greeted the patients every day at the Adelaide Street clinic. Her appearance was the occasion for a last burst of oratory and then we were asked to become serious for a moment. Esther's mother prayed in the same dignified English as the orators, for the Lord to bless her daughter and her future husband, Andrew. It was very moving and the ensuing 'amens' were fervently repeated by us all.

By this time I was extremely hungry, it was half past ten and I had only had a small piece of bread, a segment of 'Dairylea' and two cups of tea since a scanty breakfast at 7am, but deliverance was nigh. Plates of a wonderful mish-mash of different foods were being passed round, African and European, savoury and sweet, all on the same plate. It was delicious and washed down with a 'Star' was all that I wanted. Second helpings were brought round by the family and Esther circulated among the guests with her two year old daughter clinging to her leg. Her Daddy would be coming later when the dancing began and his official engagement ceremony was over.

Sylvia and I decided to slip away. As we left around midnight Esther's brother was joined by Andrew at the centre of a group of young men in the garden trying very hard to start the generator whose precious fuel had been saved for this moment, when power was needed for the cassette player and the dancing could begin.

I had received an invitation to a 'very casual' evening one Saturday from one of the wives I had met at the golf club; her husband worked up-line during the week for a tobacco company, trying to teach the local farmers how to grow it fit for export. They had a lovely twenty five year-old company house near the top of the ridge with a huge veranda overlooking Freetown and the bay which always seemed to be cooled by the breezes off the ocean. The invitation included a map but as I had not been there before I decided to do a 'recce' in the morning after I had been into town to buy stamps and a crate of Star beer for the libation on the car arranged for the next week.

Sister Cline had been very concerned by the number of punctures I had suffered, all in different circumstances and in spite of my obsessional efforts to avoid them. She assured me that this was a direct result of not having the car blessed when I first acquired it and had offered to do what was needful to put this right by presiding at a libation ceremony. Hence the beer in the boot.

The road was appalling but I reached the crest without mishap, located the compound, turned and started my descent. Near the bottom there was virtually a trench cutting diagonally across the road, I tried to drive round it and got the front off wheel impacted in a drainage ditch. Four men lifted it out and three more changed the wheel. This was my fifth puncture in three weeks. I had the inner tube patched (again) and extra padding inside the split outer tyre but I was a bit apprehensive about repeating the trip in the dark. I had been asked for 8pm and managed to arrive without incident; the ex-pats do not dine until an appreciable level of alcohol has been absorbed and we did not start eating until 10.15pm. At 1.00am I made a move and was very relieved to discover there was an alternative route down the hill by a relatively unpock-marked road, albeit the gradient was 1 in 5 in places. As I collapsed onto my bed at 1.30am I reflected that it was a good thing I had committed myself to the libation as I needed to do something to reduce the number of punctures.

On Monday before I went off to work at Wilkinson Road, I added a crate of bottled soft drinks to the box of beer in the boot and included a bottle of whisky (which I am sure had never been nearer Scotland than Nigeria) and one of rum. By 3 o'clock all the clients had gone, the registers were completed and the receipts were balanced so we were all free to enjoy the libation.

There was a serious purpose to the ceremony which was to bless my car and ask the Almighty to protect it (and me) from harm but in typical African fashion the whole procedure was carried out with so much goodwill and laughter that the occasion was a party from the start which was only partly to do with the consumption of alcohol. All the staff stood round the vehicle in a semi-circle while Sister Cline said a short prayer. Then she took the bottle of whisky (I was glad I had bought the cheapest available) and splashed it onto each wheel in turn uttering a brief blessing as the neat spirit trickled over each hub-cap. A slightly more generous libation was poured onto the roof and another onto the bonnet and the serious business was over. The remains of the whisky and all the rum were shared out in plastic cups among the senior staff and the rest shared the beer and soft drinks between them. In addition most were able to take at least one bottle of lemonade or 7-Up home with them. There was a great deal of good natured badinage about my driving skills and I gently teased Sister about the prospective efficacy of her method of protecting me from further vehicular mishaps. I never had another puncture until the week before I left Sierra-Leone for good.

I had by now a regular schedule of clinic visits which filled my week. On Mondays I went to the main clinic at Collegiate School Road, leaving at lunch time to go to the office in Adelaide Street where I would see the Director if she wished and could work on sorting out some of the many medically associated problems where my expertise was useful. These were things like supplies of drugs and instruments, keeping records, suggesting ways of improving patient flow, in-service training for our nursing staff and many other topics. A general clinic had been opened recently in the main office building, squeezed into the reception area with a minute partitioned horsebox in one corner for medical consultations and

43

examinations. This clinic was becoming increasingly popular with the local people and the clientele included not only women and their children but also older women and men.

Until my arrival this clinic, along with all the others except that at Collegiate School Road, had been run entirely by nurses. Now it was possible for them to ask any problem patients to see me either at the end of Monday morning or on Thursdays when I was there all day. I usually left about half past two or three on Mondays and called in to Collegiate on my way home in case any serious cases had turned up after the Russian doctor had left at lunch-time. This rarely happened but it enabled me to collect any drugs or dressings I needed for my last port of call before reaching home.

"You must live almost next door to the Blind School," Kelly Shepherd said to me one Thursday evening at the golf club while we were waiting our turns at the dart board.

"What Blind School?" I asked. "I have never noticed a school of any kind along my bit of Wilkinson Road."

"Of course, I forgot," she replied. "Since the Lebanese Ladies Association paid for the big wall to be put up, you can't really see it anymore, unless you're looking out for it."

I asked at the main clinic if anybody knew anything about it. They all did and were amazed at my ignorance.

"We often have children attending here," said Sister Cline. "In fact there is one waiting now."

In due course a young man with an obviously defective eye came round the curtain pushing forward a thin frightened little girl in response to the ping of my bell. She was supporting her right arm with her left.

"She fell off a top bunk at the end of last term, before she went home up-country, for her holidays. She was afraid to tell anyone as she knew she was not allowed to go on top bunks."

Her name was Faturah but she was known as Fatu. She was six years old and could understand English a little. William, who accompanied her, was, I subsequently found out, employed at the school as a general handyman and was usually the one chosen to escort the blind children as he was partially sighted.

I gently lifted the swollen arm and rested it in my hand. Midway between the wrist and elbow it was hot, red and very tender. An X-ray was obviously essential and I explained this to William. In my ignorance of the facilities I wrote a note referring the child to Connaught Hospital for the test. She came back two days later with the X-ray film and a scribbled message on the back of my note – 'Unhealed fracture of the ulna'. The Russian doctor referred her back to the hospital for treatment, as I would have done myself in those early days.

The following Monday I noticed little Fatu sitting on the end of a bench in the waiting area, tears trickling silently down her cheeks. I asked Lauretta, the SECHN (State Enrolled Community Health Nurse) to bring her in to see me straight away, before I started on the rest of the waiting room full of patients. The child was obviously in great pain and her forearm was encased completely in plaster-of-paris. I was flabbergasted; one of the cardinal rules about splinting is that a rigid plaster encircling a limb is never applied when there are signs of inflammation or swelling. No wonder she was in such pain.

Unhappily we had no plaster shears or any other means of taking off the plaster in our clinic and the only thing to do was to send her back to Connaught for its removal. I knew this would be a very painful procedure in view of the underlying swelling and inflammation. She should have had a 'back-splint' of plaster supporting the limb and held in place by, for example, a crepe bandage. She had an appointment at the hospital for later that day and I wrote a further note suggesting that as the swelling had increased overnight, it might now be advisable to remove the encircling plaster. It was no good antagonising the doctor in the hospital by expressing my opinion of his professional incompetence. Fatu was far from well and I suggested that instead of her coming back to our clinic the next day I should call in at the Blind School myself and see her there after my clinic work was finished. This was how I made my first contact with the Milton Margai School for the Blind in Freetown.

I found the school on Wilkinson Road behind its high concealing wall only five hundred yards from where I lived. I drove into the wide bare earthed forecourt where several half naked young boys were kicking a bundle of rags and paper about in lieu of a ball. They were all blind but seemed to be able to locate the 'ball' by sound alone. I parked the car and walked into a central covered passage connecting two large wooden buildings.

There were two or three benches here but as I stood rather helplessly looking to right and left uncertain which way to go, William appeared and said the Headmaster was expecting me in his office. He led me into the left hand corridor and knocked on the second door. A deep melodious voice called "Come in, come in."

It took a few seconds for my eyes to adjust to the semi-darkness after the bright tropical sunlight outside. Then I saw a good-looking man of

45

middle age standing beside his desk with hand outstretched and a very welcoming smile on his face. I explained my errand and we talked a bit. His English was impeccable and as I started explaining how the present unhappy situation had arisen and my worries about the competence of the staff at the hospital, he broke in,

"But you know we have an arrangement through VSO (Voluntary Service Overseas) with a surgeon here in private practice. He looks after any serious cases for us."

Now I'm told, I thought.

"Oh, that's excellent, we can send Fatu to see him if she is going to need specialist care. But I think perhaps I should see her now as I don't know what they did at the Connaught yesterday."

"Of course Doctor Wilson, of course. William, you take the doctor to the treatment room and bring Fatu to see her there."

I was taken back into the corridor and there almost opposite the entry was a small doorless room, dirty and dim, containing a wooden table, a bench, and a chair. William shooed out the handful of scrawny hens pecking at the bits and pieces on the floor boards. I noticed they went next door into what was obviously the dining room and found more satisfactory pickings on the tops of the trestle tables.

It was not long before Fatu arrived, her arm suspended from her neck by a dirty piece of rag as a make-do sling. This time she did have a back splint wrapped round with a grubby cotton bandage. The pain was less but she was far from comfortable. I took off the bandage without removing her arm from the splint. If anything the swelling was worse and there was no decrease in the redness. The old-fashioned mnemonic learnt by generations of medical students up to my generation (but not since I guess, as Latin was no longer required for entry to medical schools after 1950) came into my mind:-

Rubor, calor, dolor, tumor (redness, heat, pain, swelling) the classical signs of inflammation. It was therefore no surprise when William produced another crumpled bit of paper from the back pocket of his jeans with one word written on the back of my most recent note, 'Osteomyelitis?' ie infection in the bone. A second paper bore a list of eight drugs which had been prescribed, none of which included an antibiotic appropriate for treating bone infections. I had brought a crepe bandage and a sling with me from home that morning and I rebandaged her arm and used the old rag to pad the new sling where it went round the back of her neck, the nobs of her cervical vertebrae so painfully obvious in this small underweight little six year old. I supplemented her supply of paracetamol tablets (half an adult one every four hours) through William as the school had no matron or housekeeper at that time. The only resident adult female was William's eighteen year old girl friend who could be seen sitting on the bench in the passageway, bare-breasted and giving a little 'top-up' to their eighteen month old son, Abu. I decided I would like to meet Dr Ford for myself before I sent Fatu to see him. The Headmaster knew his address, which was on the way into the town centre. It was by now about 4 o'clock but a good time to catch the doctor in his hospital. I drove the two miles to Motor Main Road and found the premises without difficulty.

The door to the clinic was open and at first I could see nobody about but then an African nurse, or so I assumed her to be, appeared from behind a screen. I was not reassured by her apparel or her manner, both were extremely casual but she did inform me that the doctor was in his consulting room although he was due to go at any moment.

Fortunately Doctor Ford was a big improvement on his receptionist. He was friendly and willing to be helpful over Fatu especially as orthopaedics was his particular interest. I found out later that he did not charge the Blind School for treating their pupils but, of course, the drugs and appliances required and the costs of staying overnight in the hospital had to be met. It was not long before we were chatting like any other medical colleagues about possible mutual friends and common backgrounds. He was a Sheffield graduate of the mid-nineteen fifties and had been taught for a short time by my husband when the latter had been in charge of the Department of Therapeutics before we moved to Glasgow. He showed me round his establishment with some pride, particularly in the equipment and furnishings of the operating theatre which he had bought en-bloc from the Sheffield Regional Health Authority when the old Royal Hospital had been abandoned and all the services moved to the new Royal Hallamshire. He had had it all transhipped and here it was nearly twenty-five years later still serving a useful function. I notice there were no lights in the operating theatre and that the windows were wide open.

"I have to operate by the light of the sun," he explained. It was futile to comment on the possible contamination of open wounds by dust and minuscule debris carried in from the street outside. I realised as I became more familiar with the local situation that here was a decent man doing his best to maintain the professional standards in which he had been trained, against almost impossible odds.

We arranged that he should see Fatu at his hospital consulting room later in the week and I promised to make sure the child was started on the appropriate antibiotic, however much it would cost. We also needed to build up her strength as she was sure to be anaemic and would need some iron. Eventually little Fatu began to improve, or so we thought. She had to be re-X-rayed as the films taken at Connaught were lost somewhere in the Blind School and Dr Ford decided he would have to operate to remove what was probably a piece of dead bone from the site of the original fracture.

I took the child to the hospital in the car about 5 o'clock one Wednesday evening. She had not yet had her supper and was required to take it with her as no food was provided. As the operation was scheduled for the next morning it was all right for her to eat before six the night before. A piece of dry bread was found in the kitchen and William was sent to buy a single segment of 'Dairylea' cheese from the street seller across the road, to go with it. Holding these in her frightened little hand and clutching a very small poly-bag containing a night-dress in the other, I took her back to Motor Main Road. The omens were not auspicious; when we walked into the reception area the same indifferent nurse wandered over,

"I have brought Fatu from the Blind School, she is having an operation on her arm tomorrow," I said.

"I don't know anything about that," she replied.

"I arranged it with Dr Ford earlier in the week. Isn't Thursday his operating day?"

"Yes," she reluctantly agreed, "he probably forgot to tell me."

"Well, this is Fatu and she is completely blind, she is only six years old and has no family in Freetown. Could you at least show us where she is to sleep?" I was hoping that some embers of compassion might have been ignited by the plight of this pathetic terrified child. I might as well have been speaking to a stone wall. She was totally indifferent and it was with a heavy heart that I left the little girl curled up on her high iron bed sobbing hopelessly to herself.

Fortunately the partially-sighted wife of the VSO Field Director who taught at the school had arranged for Fatu to stay with her and her husband after the operation and was going to visit her daily. This kind and generous couple were true friends as, far from having the operation the next day, it was postponed until an anaesthetist had examined her. He was not happy with the sound of her chest and after further delays she was X-rayed and a diagnosis of tuberculosis was made. Dr Ford did an exploratory operation on her arm and decided that the lesion there was also due to TB. There was certainly no sequestrum (piece of dead bone) to remove. The treatment was medical, not surgical, and demanded daily injections of streptomycin for at least three months as well as tablets by mouth. During most of the time, while the long drawn out diagnostic procedures were being carried out, Fatu stayed with Isabelle and Richard who were fluent Krio speakers. She probably enjoyed more of the simple pleasures of childhood in those short weeks than she had experienced in the whole of her previous existence; properly fed, surrounded by TLC (tender loving care) even the pain in her arm could not swamp her happy response to what most children are given as of right.

As the end of term approached and the time came for her to go back to her family 'up-line', arrangements were made to ensure that the daily injections would continue. A VSO nurse would give them to her at a local clinic and would supervise the tablet taking.

When Fatu came back after the holidays she was obviously much worse. She had lost weight and looked like the victim of a famine, her arm was grossly swollen and gave her a great deal of very severe pain. At first this relapse was attributed to the fact that there had been some mix-up and for the last three weeks she was away she had not had her injections. The truth was more terrible. The 'tuberculous infection' in her arm had actually been an osteo-sarcoma (a very malignant tumour) which had now spread throughout her body. I had little doubt myself that what were diagnosed as multiple foci of tubercle in her chest were actually masses of tiny tumours, secondary to the primary in her arm. Even with a correct early diagnosis nothing could have been done in Sierra-Leone to save her but she might have been spared all those painful daily injections.

Towards the end of February it was apparent that Fatu was dying and her parents took her back to their village up-country. They made a last effort to save her by calling on the resources of the local medicine-man. She was held in the smoke of burning leaves and other magic ingredients and died of asphyxia which at least cut short her sufferings by a few days. Apart from giving her supplies of paracetamol which were totally ineffective for much of her illness, my intervention had done nothing to postpone her death and had done a lot to increase her suffering with unnecessary investigations, an operation and weeks of injections.

Nan was from Liberia. She had escaped with her two children from Monrovia, the capital, and was staying with a distant relative in Freetown. She was a trained nurse and was employed on a temporary contract by

Marie-Stopes. She was competent but moody and rarely smiled. This was not surprising as she and the children had to sleep on the kitchen floor and she found sharing a very small house with her second cousin and her second cousin's husband and three children very difficult. She had not heard from her husband since she left Liberia four months before. Even so, the other West Africans with whom I worked showed a remarkable resilience in the face of adversity and smiled and laughed both with clients and among themselves. Nan was always tired, which can be a symptom of depression, but then she began complaining of headaches and I started wondering if there was more to her ill-health than the stresses of living as a refugee.

"Have you ever had a problem with your blood pressure?" I asked her. She was only twenty nine but hypertension is very common in West Africa.

"Oh no Doctor Wilson, I am very healthy."

I knew the poor woman was desperate to keep her job and would have given herself a medical history free of any suggestion of chronic illness.

"That's fine but I think I'll just check it now, you really don't seem to be completely fit."

With some reluctance she allowed me to wrap the sphygmo-manometer cuff round her upper arm. I kept my face expressionless as I pumped the air into the cuff under increasing resistance. I was inwardly dismayed to find that the reading was 210/160, the upper limit of the normal range being 130/90 given the stress of having it taken. I repeated the whole procedure. Nan was no fool and she could read the figure herself when she felt the blood pulsing through. She looked at me in misery.

"You've had some degree of high blood pressure for some time haven't you?" I asked her gently.

"Yes," she reluctantly admitted. "It was high in both my pregnancies and never went down after the last."

"How old is that baby now?"

"He's nearly three, but Doctor I've got to keep this job. I've no money otherwise and if I can't pay my cousin we'll be thrown out on the street and we'll have to go to a camp out of town and I'll never get a job again."

"There's no need to say anything to anybody else at present but you need treatment urgently. As a member of staff you get your drugs free if we have them in stock, you know that. I'll prescribe the tablets you need and then I'll check your blood pressure again next week and see how it's responded."

I knew that it would be impossible to keep her health problem a secret as all the prescriptions were checked against the receipts and those for staff were kept on one side and added to the total. It was essential to keep a very tight control on drug supplies. The girl who did the checking would know at once that Nan was suffering from hypertension and it would be all round the office almost before I had written my signature. However, if her condition improved and she was able to do her work competently, it should not affect her prospects.

The following week there was some improvement but not as much as I had hoped.

"Have you been taking the tablets regularly? You're sure you haven't forgotten any?"

"Oh no, Doctor Wilson but I have been so worried about my brother."

"Your brother? You haven't mentioned him before!"

"He's only just got here from Liberia and his arms are paralysed. He's here now in the waiting room. Would you see him? He's frightened he'll never be able to work." Nan went out and returned holding a thin undernourished young man by his upper arm.

"Hello, your Nan's brother are you? What's your name?"

His sister answered for him, "David Green."

"You look as though you've had a bad time. What happened to you?"

This time he answered for himself and like his sister and most other Liberians, his English was good.

"I was working in a small town outside Monrovia when I heard the rebels were coming so I tried to run away, to come to Sierra-Leone where I knew my sister had come. At first I managed to hitch a lift and I found enough fruits to eat round the villages but then the soldiers came and caught me. I thought I would be shot but they put me in a truck with many others and tied my arms behind my back very tight. We were not untied for two days and a night. One of the other prisoners was allowed to give us a drink of water in the morning and at night time; we had to sleep on the ground with our arms tied but I was in so much pain I could not. Then for no reason they let us go, we were near Zimmi so it was not so far to get over the border but then I had to walk to Freetown and my hands are not working."

"Would you take off your shirt please, I want to examine you?" I requested, deliberately leaving him to do it himself so that I could assess how severely he was disabled. His left arm hung down and was slightly twisted so that his curved fingers and palm faced outwards as though waiting to receive an unsanctioned tip, but with encouragement it became apparent that although he had undoubtedly suffered a partial brachial nerve palsy on both sides, the left being the most severe, it was already recovering. He managed to get his shirt off once his sister had undone the buttons. Although the injuries had been inflicted over three weeks before, the rope marks on his upper arms were very evident. The skin must have been cut into and the wounds had become infected although they had now healed and only the scars and the nerve damage remained as evidence of what he had been through. He had been afraid to move his arms in case he made them worse but I reassured him.

"The ropes pressed on the nerves that go to the muscles in your arms and hands. The nerves were bruised and couldn't work properly so you could not move your muscles; the bruising also made you feel pins and needles in your hands and took away some of the feeling but you know yourself you are already getting better. I don't want you to rest your arms and hands, I want you to exercise them. Grip this," I held out the rolled up notebook I used in which to keep a record of my petrol consumption.

"You see you can hold that quite well with your right hand, not so good with your left. Now put it down and I want you to try and grip this piece of paper between the tips of your thumb and each finger in turn."

It was difficult to see if there was any true muscle wasting because both hands had been affected and he was very thin. I thought there was a good chance of complete recovery. He had been a healthy seventeen year old before his encounter with the rebels and I suppose had been lucky not to have suffered more or been press-ganged into becoming yet another trigger-happy young revolutionary. He was almost certainly anaemic from the look of his conjunctiva when I gently pulled down his lower lid to assess its pinkness. He had probably got worms and his sister would certainly have no faith in my treatment and the prognosis for his brachial injuries unless I prescribed an injection of Vitamin B Co to restore his strength. So young David went out with worm pills, iron tablets, vitamin preparations and a puncture wound in his backside in which he had more faith than any of my words about exercising his limbs.

The next week he returned looking a lot better and with much improved power and feeling in his hands. At the end of a month he had almost recovered except for a little weakness in his left grip. As he was registered with the Red Cross as a refugee his treatment was free and he had a regular rice ration. He was already looking for work.

I had been having my weekly shampoo and set one Saturday morning in preparation for a meal with the Emerys at the British High Commission that evening. I said goodbye to Vivienne in her little salon at the back of the Cape Sierra Hotel and walked along the corridor to the top of the stairs which led down into the main concourse with the bar on the right at the back. There I stopped, looking down with a mixture of dismay and fascination at the scene below me. It was a press conference. Twenty or more journalists or media men, some with cameras, were faced by at least a dozen of the most fearsome looking bandits I had ever seen, even on a television screen.

Most wore filthy jeans but these were the only attempt at uniformity. Some had animal skins tied by the legs over one shoulder, a few wore combat jackets that looked like the ragged remains of army uniforms but most bizarre of all were two men who had old western type women's dresses that reached to mid-calf, on top of their T-shirts and trousers. Their headgear was equally unconventional. Two wore female European style wigs, one a squashed top hat but the most popular headgear were baseball caps worn back to front. Those whose arms were bare had a tattoo below the shoulder which I found out later was a skull and cross-bones. They were all armed and most were leaning against a wall or draped round the non-functioning television set carelessly cradling Kalashnikovs.

The central figure, who appeared to be taller than the rest, had a leopard skin over his shoulders and was addressing the audience with a strong American accent. This was Prince Johnson, the third party in the Liberian civil war. He had started off as a member of Charles Taylor's rebels but had fallen out with him and set up his own independent army. He had flown in from Monrovia to put his case to the World's press, or at least the very small part of it which was in Freetown to meet him. He appeared to be getting annoyed by some of the questions and his bodyguard did not look like men who would be worried by the death of a passer-by if she were caught in the crossfire. I slipped quickly and quietly down the stairs and went out through the nearest door.

The news from Liberia of President Doe's death had came as no surprise and no tears were shed. He had been a savage and ruthless dictator and rumours abounded of his brutality. I was told by two different people whose word I respected that he would gnaw the amputated finger of a political enemy during meetings, much as others might chew gum or munch peanuts. Once he was delivered into rebel hands he was shown no mercy and died a terrible death. He was mutilated while still alive by having pieces of his body cut off over a period of several hours until he died from shock and exsanguination. These barbarities were compounded by being recorded on video camera. The tape was on sale in Freetown within a week and I met several people subsequently who had seen it. They were not people I respected. To watch this atrocity while sitting in a comfortable armchair sipping a gin and tonic seemed to me to be participating vicariously, to be totally lacking in any civilised values, without even the hate and anger which must have motivated the torturers.

There were more uplifting stories that came out of Monrovia. One concerned the sole remaining British embassy official who stayed on in the building with six dogs which had had to be left behind by their evacuated owners. There were no British troops to guard him but he not only managed to survive, he also took a truck to rescue what was left of a mission school, hospital or orphanage – versions varied. The inhabitants were starving and more than half had died before he reached them but the rest he brought back and handed over to the Americans for medical help and evacuation.

Chapter 3 – October
Is That Your Boy Friend, Doctor?

IT WAS THURSDAY AROUND 4 O'CLOCK.
I could not face the thought of another dark sweating night, preceded by a sardine sandwich washed down with warm Sprite.

Jane and Donald lived in a lovely house high on the ridge above the city and I had often enjoyed delicious vegetarian meals followed by Pavarotti or a good film on video, under their roof. They had given me an open invitation to 'drop in' at any time and now I felt the time had arrived. It was not, of course, possible to warn them of my impending arrival but I was not really worried about my welcome.

There were several different routes I could choose from. But in practice, I nearly always went up the looping curves of Spur Road, left at the top for half a mile when the more or less tarmaced surface petered out and red mud and pot-holes marked the rest of the track. Not far from their compound there was a large refuse skip into which the local households tossed their rubbish to be emptied fairly regularly by the city authorities. As I crawled past I saw a large black snake (dead) well over six feet long, hanging over the side of the skip so I stopped to have a better look. I think it was probably a spitting cobra which is common enough in the gardens of dwellers on the hills. While I was stationary a very small and almost hairless puppy crawled out from behind the skip. It was so weak it could hardly move. Stray and abandoned dogs are so common in Sierra-Leone that I am afraid I barely noticed it. I drove up to the gates of the compound, was recognised by the watchmen and was allowed in, to be greeted rumbustiously by Jane's assorted menagerie. The two dogs, one with a stiff hind leg which she had set and splinted when she found him lying injured in the road, the other blind in one eye; the small cat who had been born with useless forelimbs and the other who was adult but the size of a kitten; the monkey in its large bell-shaped cage, left behind by returning expatriates, who had had it from infancy tethered by a belt and chain which had produced a ring of sores

55

round her body – all these helpless creatures had been lovingly nursed back to health and looked after from then on.

I had a fellow feeling with these disadvantaged orphans as I too was looking for food and shelter from these two warm and generous friends. Jane welcomed me and sat me down on their open veranda with a cold drink to enjoy the breeze from the ocean – the ocean which stretched away to the horizon beyond the huddle of houses, the nine-hole golf course and the palm-fringed beach, until it reached America. The ground sloped steeply and I was able to watch a great variety of birds in the tree canopy alongside and below the level of the veranda.

We waited for Donald to come home from the mill and then enjoyed a truly delicious vegetarian dinner. Jane did all her own cooking which was unusual among the Europeans. She also went out of her way, literally, to buy really fresh vegetables. She knew a small market gardener in a village in the hinterland behind Freetown who grew carrots, onions and tomatoes as well as many other 'fruits in their season'. She washed them all well in Milton solution which certainly appeared to be effective as neither I, nor any other partaker at her table, ever suffered any ill consequences.

After we had eaten Donald said, "Why don't you stay the night? I'm sure we can find you some night attire and it seems silly to go back to darkness and no air-conditioning when you can stay here."

It was an offer I was far too weak-minded to refuse. I thankfully relaxed and was able to enjoy *Some Like it Hot* knowing I did not have to face the awkward drive back and the hazards of unlit enormous trucks parked halfway across Wilkinson Road where the on-coming vehicles always drove with undipped lights. Next morning was Saturday and not my turn to do the main clinic so there was no rush to get moving.

"It would be really nice if you could stay over the weekend. We are planning to go to Tokay Beach tomorrow, you've never been have you?" asked Jane.

I went back to the flat in daylight and collected all I was likely to need and gratefully returned to my hospitable haven. On Sunday morning we set off for Tokay Beach, Donald was driving and as we neared the skip I remembered the puppy. As soon as I began talking about it I wondered whether I should have kept my mouth shut as it was inevitable that Jane's tender heart would not allow her to disregard its piteous plight. I secretly hoped it would either be dead or gone but there it was, barely able to stand, panting in the heat. Nobody said anything more and we drove past and talked of other things. It only took about forty minutes to get to the Beach in the air-conditioned four-wheel drive vehicle. We parked in the shade of the hotel forecourt and wandered through the reception area and out onto the white sand fringing the deep blue Atlantic. We found a wooden sunbed each and relaxed in the partial shade of a palm thatched umbrella. African waiters came to enquire what we would like to drink and presented us with menus in French for lunch. This was, in fact, a French owned and French run establishment and most of the guests, certainly all the residents, were French also. It was expensive by Sierra-Leonian standards but not by European.

We were content to have beer and cheese sandwiches brought to our chaise-longues, but not until after we had plunged into the sea. The beach shelved but not steeply and the rollers were big but not overwhelming and it was bliss to lie on the surface and be lifted up and in, be dropped gently on the shifting sand, swim gently out and do it again. It was the first time I had bathed in the sea since I had visited my sister in Australia six years before. I hate swimming in cold water and hate even more trying to dry myself with an inadequate towel in a damp confined cubicle with the smell of chlorine pricking my nostrils while trying to avoid dropping my swimsuit onto the floor among other peoples' hairs and dirty sticking plasters. If, in addition, one is fat with rolls of flab, and the pendulous parts of one's anatomy are normally confined within the contours of a corselet, one is reluctant to expose the true horrors to public gaze. Only the tropical sea can motivate me enough to strip off and squeeze into my swim-suit, even though it does have a discrete little skirt across the bottom of the front panel. On this occasion I was encouraged by the horrendous sight of elderly adipose French persons of both sexes exposing all but a minuscule triangle of their naked flesh to the view of anybody misguided enough to look at it.

We left for home about 4 o'clock and were nearly back on the 'main' (unsurfaced) track when we had to stop as there were two vehicles stopped in front of us. The road was wide enough for us to pass had they both been on the same side but each stayed obstinately facing each other on opposite sides with two or three yards between them. It is no use getting upset about the passage of time in Africa. We watched fascinated as the two drivers got out and began an apparently angry altercation. As time passed others began to emerge from the two clapped-out old bangers and added their views to the argument until at least nine people were standing between the cars shaking their heads and waving their arms about. Eventually agreement seemed to have been reached and we thought we would soon be on our way.

But no, to our amazement, two of the men half disappeared into the back of one of the vehicles and, after a great deal of heaving and struggling, pulled out a reluctant goat and transferred it into the other car. The drivers and passengers all got back inside (although how this was possible without suffocating the goat it was hard to imagine) and drove off. The episode had taken nearly fifteen minutes but, for me, it was time well spent, although not, I think, in Donald's opinion – he still had a rough and tedious drive in front of him.

When we were nearly home he stopped the car by the skip and Jane got out. The puppy was still alive, just. His body was covered in sores and he was so emaciated that his skin stretched over his ribs like cling-film. Jane scooped him up and cupping him easily in her hands, she brought him home. She treated him for ticks, ring-worm and every possible external and internal parasite from tapeworms to fleas, and he had them all. She fed him and he ate and ate and his bulging abdomen nearly touched the ground until his little stumpy legs started to grow and so did the rest of him. She loved him and the rest of the menagerie accepted him. I was the only one with subsequent reservations, when, three months later, he would bound up to me with unrestrained fervour and lovingly push his enormous paws on my chest as I got out of the car, whether it had just been raining or not.

Wednesday was my day at King Tom and Aberdeen. I set off at a quarter to eight, picking up one or two girls whose schools lay on my route. I soon learnt to recognise the different uniforms of the girls' secondary schools, there are very few mixed educational establishments in Freetown. By leaving early I usually managed to avoid the worst of the traffic and was able to drive in third or fourth gear for at least the first mile. The importance of this lay not so much in the waste of time involved in driving at less than fifteen miles per hour but in the need to conserve petrol. By keeping records of fuel consumption and mileage I was able to show that I could save over a gallon of petrol a week by going early and driving in a high gear rather than grinding along, stopping and starting and never moving out of third.

Soon the vehicles from the feeder roads increased the congestion so that one was forced into first or second approaching the Congo Main Road roundabout. It was here that the Peugeot Estates, the Mercedes and the big four-wheel drive Japanese convertibles from the American Embassy compound and the wealthy mansions on the crest of the hill filtered their way into the main stream traffic with the active collusion of the duty policeman. It always surprised me that after the next congested half mile the traffic suddenly thinned out and we all speeded up.

Then, as I waited at the lights (which were often working as they were outside the government Department of Health) I noticed a girl, no more than six years old, thread her way through the waiting vehicles. She carried a half full five gallon water drum in one hand, a bulging plastic bag in the other and balanced on her head was an inverted wooden stool with a tray of shoe cleaning things resting between its legs. She was smiling cheerfully and gave me a grin as she waited on the island for the lights to change.

Once on the road to the King Tom police barracks there were no more hold-ups but I made my customary diversion to the Red Lion bakery where I could buy fresh white bread. On Saturdays, if I was not working and arrived early enough, one could also get brown or even a malt loaf. However, I was content on a weekday, with having a loaf rather than the usual rolls as this bread kept better for the next day. I reached the barracks about a quarter past eight and decided to explore the Commonwealth War Grave Cemetery which was adjacent. It is a beautiful and peaceful place with a huge cotton tree guarding its sleeping occupants. There are few houses in the immediate vicinity, the access road carries little traffic and the side bounded by the sea affords no access to the public – officially that is. Admittedly the stand-pipe in the centre of the graveyard was obviously being used by some people to do their washing but they left no mess and only the trampled grass and foot-imprinted mud betrayed their recent presence. Most of the memorials were of the standard first or second world war pattern, plain stones rounded at the top bearing the name, date and service rank of the dead. Many carried touching messages to beloved sons, husbands and fathers.

I was poignantly aware that most of those who had chosen their heartfelt thoughts to be inscribed were now themselves remembered only as names perhaps by elderly grandchildren.

Many graves were of sailors in the Merchant Navy who had died, not in battle but of sickness. Sierra-Leone had been known as 'The White Man's Grave', but the biggest killer had not been malaria or yellow fever but the 'Spanish flu' which had spread like a forest fire through the tight-packed mess decks of cargo ships in 1918 and 19. There are others buried there who had served the old Empire in colonial days and died in time of peace. There is for example, a woman missionary who died in her forties after years of service. It seemed to me entirely fitting that these others should be included in this essentially English Cemetery and that the relatives of those other combatants with whom we were at war at the time of their deaths would feel that they too were at peace even in such an alien land.

Sic transit gloria mundi; it was a good job I had to start work and was unable to indulge in any further melancholy thoughts.

The King Tom clinic was held in a concrete cell nine feet square with a door, an unglazed window, a tall cupboard, an examination couch, a table, two chairs and a small stand on which the instruments, gloves etc necessary for gynaecological examinations were set out. Regina collected the water required for washing my hands in a bowl from a stand-pipe fifty yards away. The patients waited outside in a covered porch on a concrete bench. Most of them were women, some for family planning, some ante-natal and some with problems of infertility, irregular bleeding, lower abdominal pain and so on. This police barracks had a daily medical clinic which wives and children might attend but whose medical officer was only too happy for Marie-Stopes to see 'female problems'.

The first patient was a woman in European dress who spoke good English. She was a twenty four year old school teacher, who had been married for two years and was concerned about her fertility.

"Have you had any pregnancies before?" I asked her.

"Yes," she replied, "I had an abortion when I was seventeen. I was still at school and if I had had the baby I couldn't have finished my studies."

It was a common enough story but when I examined her vaginally everything felt completely normal.

"Were you ill after the abortion? Did you have a fever? Were you given any antibiotics?"

"No, I was only about nine weeks and it only took ten minutes."

Sister quietly intervened, "Who was the doctor who did the operation?"

I had met the named doctor at an international symposium in Europe a year before and had enjoyed a very pleasant evening as her guest in her beautiful house in Freetown with its fabulous views over the ocean. I knew she ran a lucrative private practice but so did all the other doctors in Freetown if they had the ability to do so.

Sister Meux pulled me over gently to the window and murmured, "This doctor always inserts an I.U.D when she does a termination and she doesn't usually tell the girl, especially if the parents ask her not to."

This suggestion made me examine the woman again to make quite certain that I could neither feel nor see any trace of nylon filaments protruding through the opening in the cervix uteri. There were none. I had explained to her why I was checking her again and suggested sending her for an ultra-sound scan which would show whether a 'coil' was present or not. It was only recently that the consultant radiologist had acquired both the machine and the skill needed to use it, which was a great bonus in cases like the present. An X-ray of the pelvis would also demonstrate the device but could cause serious damage to the foetus if the women did happen to be in the early weeks of pregnancy and a scan would be preferable. I carefully tore a clean sheet of A4 paper into six pieces, Sister stamped the clinic name on the top of one of the bits with the purple ink stamp, I wrote the patient's name and age and put:-

'Two years infertility? I.U.D. in situ. U.S.S. (ultra sound scan) pelvis, please.' I signed and dated it, folded it over and wrote the name of the radiologist and the address of his rooms on one side. It was important to leave enough space on the paper for the report as this was always scribbled on the request note which the patient brought back with her. When I first worked in Sierra-Leone I used to follow the British practice:–

'Dear Dr Whosit, Mrs XYZ d.o.b. 3.6.46. Please would you see this patient who is complaining of . . . . . . for the last six years. O.E. (on examination) I can find no abnormality and would be grateful for your opinion. With kind regards (if I knew him personally) Yours sincerely.'

In Africa there was neither the time nor the paper to indulge in these professional courtesies and one only referred patients to someone else if an essential investigation was needed or some procedure required for which we did not have the facilities, such as surgery, rehydration therapy for severely dehydrated babies or predicted complications of labour. I do not think our patients suffered in Freetown because of the brevity of the communications between colleagues, but I quickly became aware that it was even more important than in the UK to know the calibre of the doctor to whom the person was referred. The other major factor was whether the patient had the money to pay for whatever was needed. If they had not, that was just too bad and they died or recovered without the intervention of Western medicine. Native treatments also cost money but did not appear to be as expensive as that provided by qualified doctors although they were sometimes extremely painful, mutilating and unsuccessful.

Fortunately there was no need to be concerned about this lady's ability to pay as she was not only working herself but her husband had a reasonably well paid job and was as anxious as she was to have the problem sorted out. They were Christian Krios and there was no question of him taking a second wife if this one did not produce a child.

The following Wednesday she was already waiting when Sister arrived to open the clinic. She was an intelligent woman and had read the brief report 'I.U.D. in place'. Of course this merely confirmed the suspected diagnosis and I still had to try and remove the device, which would not be easy without the threads to get hold of. However, I had had a great deal of experience with this problem and had prepared for the situation by bringing with me from the main clinic a sterile instrument with a long handle rather like a crochet hook. This tool had never been used as no-one knew what it was for. I confess to some personal satisfaction as I gently inserted the slim blunt hook, rotated it through 360 degrees and pulled it towards me. I could feel that there was some resistance but continued the firm but gentle traction. As the instrument was withdrawn from the os (the opening into the uterus through the cervix) it brought with it the end of a nylon thread. After that it was a simple matter to grip the end with a pair of artery forceps and pull. The Lippes Loop came out sweetly and easily much to the delight of all of us – the patient, the doctor, the sister and the nursing aid, all crammed into a little concrete box, nine feet by nine in a temperature of 90 degrees and humidity at 92 percent.

About a quarter to eleven Sister Meux asked Regina to get my cup of tea. She always went outside for at least ten minutes and would then appear carefully carrying a very full mug of scalding hot pale straw coloured liquid into which she would stir at least three heaped teaspoonfuls of powdered milk. I had managed to convince her that I did not take sugar after the first occasion when no less than four lumps had been added, but I did not want to appear too critical and so made no remonstrance over the milk. Indeed, I found the mixture quite refreshing and palatable as long as I did not think of it as tea. I saw my last patient while my steaming mug cooled and then departed leaving Sister to see the remaining ante-natal patients.

I was due next at the Aberdeen clinic. This was held every Wednesday in the local police station. I looked forward to this session, the drive there from King Tom was usually trouble free and lay through largely residential suburbs before Aberdeen Ferry Road took me across the long bridge spanning the shallow inlet onto the peninsula, almost an island, on which Aberdeen village was situated. The trees and shrubby vegetation concealed the size of the township but it was large enough to justify having its own police station which was sited a little apart from the village proper in the open ground that lay around the three major hotels.

The small building was hexagonal with the reception desk in the central area, which fronted a wide opening, flanked by a veranda on each side. Our clinic was held in the left hand segment which was separated from the central area by a wall about four feet high supplemented by a blue curtain to fill in the open space above. Our receptionist sat at a table inside the 'hall'. The women, many with one or more children, sat on a bench beside the reception table and the overflow waited on the veranda. There was no privacy at reception but as they nearly all knew each other and were probably neighbours this was of no importance to the clients. Similarly all the individuals who were complaining to, or being questioned by, the police had to do it all in public, and very noisy they were on some occasions so that there was, in practice, a relatively high degree of confidentiality once the patient was through the door and behind the blue curtain.

On this Wednesday a woman was sobbing loudly, and shouting abuse about someone, probably her husband who had beaten her up. Her injuries were not sufficiently severe to warrant medical attention according to the sergeant who was trying to make sense of her complaint. The uproar continued for nearly an hour, and one of the toddlers started crying in sympathy, or perhaps fright. Even without today's extra decibels there was always a background chatter of people laughing and talking and the intermittent bleating of the goats as they foraged round the outside of the building for some more succulent blades of grass.

Gradually I came to recognise the 'regulars', among them two elderly women, one of the young policemen and several mothers who brought one or other of their children nearly every week. One of the old ladies had a large benign goitre but fortunately this did not bother her as she would never have been able to afford an operation to remove it. Her problems were those of elderly people the world over, cough, pains in her knees and in West Africa, a raised blood pressure. It was not very high and I decided to say nothing about it as effective treatment would be life-long and the cost of the anti-hypertensive tablets would reduce her meagre income significantly. The knowledge that it was raised would only be a source of anxiety and would entail yet more visits to the clinic. However, diuretics are cheap and certainly help and she could afford to take two tablets a day on Mondays, Wednesdays and Fridays 'to strengthen the heart'.

Listening to the chest with a stethoscope was an important part of the reassurance which patients expected from the doctor and I always did so whether I thought it was really necessary or not. In many ways my age was a clinical advantage as I had been a medical student before the days of most of the high tech aids to diagnosis which are taken for granted today. Apart from X-rays and simple ECGs we had to rely on our four senses – at least the use of the fifth had been discontinued by 1949 – we no longer tasted the urine. Observation was paramount and preceded even the formal examination. How did the patient walk into the room, what was his or her demeanour, manner of sitting down, facial expression, general appearance, obvious abnormalities? These were what we were trained to look for.

Old Mrs Karomah walked slowly in to the room using a stick and lowered herself gingerly onto the chair holding on to the corner of the table with her free hand. She looked a little anxious but was obviously not in pain except when she was in the act of sitting down. She had been a tall woman before arthritis made her stoop over her stick and must have been a fine looking lady in her youth and middle age. She was not fat but not skinny either and had obviously not had any significant weight loss in the recent past. Once settled in the chair she gave me a warm smile and said, "It's me cough, Doctor and me knees."

Use of one's ears was the second most important faculty and, again, came into play before the stethoscope was applied. The patient's voice could tell one a lot, especially if it was not normal, huskiness could be transient and due to a sore throat but over a longer time might be more sinister and indicate malignancy. Sometimes the person's breathing was audible, it might be wheezy or laboured; a patient with a cough would almost certainly make sure that the doctor was given an unsolicited demonstration even before the shirt was removed; a hard dry cough indicates a different diagnosis from a loose phlegmy one. Mrs Karomah, on cue, duly coughed into a fold of her lappa-lappa.

"It keep me awake night time, I can't sleep."

"Do you cough anything up?"

"Sometime, small small," she replied.

"Have you coughed up blood?"

"No, no, nothing like that."

The nurse, knowing the drill, helped me pull up the old lady's upper garment and I applied my stethoscope. There were the expected noises indicating a mild chest infection but no signs of pneumonia or severe bronchitis. She was too well in herself for either of those more serious conditions.

"Now what about your knees?" I enquired.

She pulled up her voluminous wrap-round skirt and exposed two misshapen joints obviously distorted by the effects of osteoarthritis. I took her foot (minus its thonged sandal) into my hand and gently extended her lower leg and flexed it back again while I rested my other hand on the swollen joint. As I had expected I could feel the crepitations as the rough ends of the bones moved over one another but it was not really painful and there are no knee replacements available in Sierra-Leone at a price this old lady could afford.

"Ma, I can't give you new knees but I'll give you panadol for when they ache. You have small problem in your chest, not serious but you need ampicillin for that and I'll give you tablets to help you sleep until the antibiotic cures your cough."

The urban population of Freetown is relatively sophisticated in its knowledge of drugs, at least they are familiar with the names and functions of those that are easily available as no prescription is necessary and the only barrier is their cost. I had to remember to use the trade name and not the generic or scientific name, hence 'paracetamol' was always 'panadol' to nurses and patients alike. Dispensing our own supply of drugs was an important part of a clinic's function and in the smaller peripheral sessions the consulting room table was half covered with an assortment of jars and bottles containing supplies of chloroquine, vitamins, panadol, phenergan, iron tablets, septrin, ampicillin capsules, tablets against worms – thread, round, tape, hook, – lasix, the only diuretic we stocked; inderal our sole anti-hypertensive agent and large bottles of benzyl-benzoate lotion for the treatment of scabies. This is not an exhaustive list but gives some idea of the most commonly prescribed treatments.

Patients attending the Marie-Stopes clinics paid a consultation fee which covered them for a month so that they would not be discouraged from follow-up visits that might be medically needed, by having to pay every time they attended. The amount, by European standards, was very small and even for employed adults was never more than 75p. Fees for children under five and those over sixty were only about 30p and ante-natal patients also paid a very reduced rate. Family planning patients were heavily subsidised and paid about 50p for a year regardless of how many times they came. All patients paid for the drugs and appliances they were prescribed and, although these were a fraction of what they would have been charged by the commercial pharmacies, the total cost was often more than the amount they had brought with them. Sometimes it was possible for them to pay for the most urgently needed preparation, for example half a bottle of ampicillin syrup for a small baby with a severe chest infection, and then arrange to return later with the rest of the money for the other items after their husband had returned from work with some more cash. At other times there was apparently no possibility of further supplies.

"Show me what you got," Sister would demand and the patient would unclutch her fingers from a filthy role of bank notes, none of which was worth more than 5p. These would be laboriously added up.

"Not enough," Sister would relentlessly state. "Come on, I know you have more, you'd better show me all." The reluctant woman would then fumble at her waist where the fold of her skirt was tucked in to hold it up. The corner of the material would be knotted on itself and when eventually undone a further supply of higher denomination notes would be revealed. As quick as a striking cobra Sister's hand would be in there, snatching the bundle and counting out what sum was needed to pay for the drugs.

"You must not be too soft, Doctor. I know this woman, her husband has a good job in the Red Lion Bakery but she knows Marie-Stopes is funded from abroad and she thinks she can get her treatment for nothing." So Sister explained her apparently hard-hearted persistence.

Happily Mrs Karomah was not one of those who tried to evade paying and she had enough leones with her to pay for the tablets she needed. I counted them out; ampicillin capsules, two, three times a day for three days – eighteen altogether at ten leones each, this was by far the most expensive item but also the most necessary; ten panadol, two to be taken when needed, one leone each; ten phenergan, two each night, (I hoped the antibiotic would cure the cough before they ran out) at two leones each; and lastly the diuretic which might help to clear her chest if there was a cardiac component in it, as well as help her hypertension, two in the morning on Monday, Wednesday and Friday for two weeks. The whole lot cost less than a British pound but it was as much as she could afford.

Each collection of tablets was placed in the centre of a rectangular piece of paper, usually used A4, typed on one side but no longer needed by the office. Each sheet was torn into three and sometimes the strips were further subdivided. Ten phenergan could easily be parcelled up in a sixth of a sheet of old typing paper but the ampicillin capsules were much bulkier and needed half a sheet to contain them safely. Mrs Karomah could read but there was no room to write wordy instructions on the little packets. We marked each in pencil with the appropriate number of vertical strokes arranged accordingly – ampicillin II II II, phenergan II, etc and hoped that she would remember that they were to help her sleep and should be taken at night.

My weekly sessions at Aberdeen police station were to prove useful in the future when a professional contact with the local police could have been difficult if they had not learnt to trust me.

One Thursday evening at the golf club I was partnered at darts by a well built young man in his mid-thirties. He told me he was getting married in the near future and his fiancée was flying out from England for the ceremony. I was amazed.

"Has she been out here before?" I asked him.

"Oh no, it'll be her first time. The trouble is we've had a bit of bother with the flight out. I'd planned for her to be here for a week beforehand but now it looks as though she'll be arriving the night before."

"Well," I said. "She probably won't mind that much, as long as the ferry is running to Lungi and you will be there to meet her at the airport."

"Yes, but you see, I haven't told her and the wedding is on Saturday!"

Interesting, I thought, but perhaps if she is game enough to come out to Freetown to be married she will take the concertinaed arrangements in her stride.

"I suppose you wouldn't like to come would you?" he added rather diffidently. "The more the merrier, you know."

I wondered whether he really meant it but his aim at the dart board was ten times as accurate as mine and he was only on his third 'Star' of the night.

"Are you sure? I only met you for the first time last week."

"Positive, we Brits have got to stick together you know. It's in the Registrar's Office in Laminah Sankoh Street at 11 o'clock and then there's a buffet lunch at the Marine Club afterwards."

I accepted with alacrity. I always enjoyed new experiences and the thought of such an interesting morning followed by nice food in pleasant surroundings with the opportunity to meet friends and acquaintances was not to be missed.

On Saturday morning I found the Registrar's office with some difficulty. Laminah Sankoh Street is only about five hundred yards long and has decaying Government offices down one side so it should have been easy. I had been looking for something more imposing than the reality, an inconspicuous doorway between shop-fronts with a small faded door plaque announcing the presence of the Registrar's Office upstairs.

Three floors up a dirty narrow staircase there was a corridor with a long wooden bench under an unglazed barred window. I gratefully collapsed onto the seat, hot, sticky and breathless after the climb. As usual I was the first there but was soon joined by other wedding guests. We sat or stood in the dusty passage awaiting the arrival of the main protagonists.

After twenty minutes the bridegroom could be heard progressing jovially up the stairs escorted by several supporters (all male, of course). The Registrar then appeared from an adjacent office and let us into the marriage chamber. She was a very elegant Sierra-Leonian lady wearing a jade green outfit and gold earrings and necklace who conducted the ensuing ceremony with dignity and friendliness in spite of the unpropitious surroundings. What had once been a fairly large room had been divided by a false wall and at least half the remaining space was occupied by a large table. There was just enough room for her to sit behind it and for the bridal pair to face her flanked by the best man and matron of honour. The rest of the party squashed onto the single row of chairs lining the walls. The windows were free of glass and the noises from the street and of an air-conditioner in some more fortunate adjacent office made the acoustics difficult. The dirt encrusted vanes of a similar but long unused air-conditioner were a sad reminder of more prosperous times. The wall opposite the window was lined with a book case filled with enormous tomes and ledgers none of which bore a date later than 1932.

We had plenty of time in which to observe all these details as it was a further fifteen minutes before the bride arrived and all was ready. The Registrar began by reading out the legal requirements on the consenting parties as laid down in a statute of, I think, 1894. The fine for giving false information was five leones (the rate of exchange was currently 300 to the pound sterling). We all sat solemnly poker-faced while this archaic piece of legal jargon was completed and then it was quickly followed by the more familiar words of the marriage ceremony as exported from England throughout the British Empire. It did not take long and both bride and groom were obviously relieved when they could relax and he was able to take off the grey jacket of his suit which was wet through from shoulder to shoulder in the heat and humidity of that overcrowded room.

The tension over, the whole party joined in with congratulations and there was a genuine air of happy hilarity which was in marked contrast to the dreary surroundings. We all clattered down the stairs and made our way out of the town to the Marine Club to enjoy the wedding breakfast under the palms on the edge of Lumley beach.

I never saw that generous young man again as he left the country for good shortly afterwards but I shall always be grateful to him for including me among his wedding guests.

Tuesday was the day I went in the Land-Rover with Sister Meux, Keturah and one of the other SECH nurses on our weekly trip to Hastings, Jui, and Grafton. As we drove round the Up-Gun roundabout onto the main road out of the city we were overtaken by Ken Shepherd whom I had met with his wife at the golf club, driving himself, as usual, in his ODA (Overseas Development Administration) Land-Rover. He gave a toot and a wave and quickly out-distanced our elderly vehicle.

"Is that your boy friend Doctor?" Sister Meux asked slyly. The other nurses added their comments,

"I've seen you wave to him before," said Keturah.

"Of course," I replied. "I am having a passionate affair with him. No, seriously, he and his wife have been very kind to me and they are both good friends of mine." This explanation did not prevent a lot of good natured ribbing whenever the ODA Land-Rover was sighted with its diagnostic Union Jack painted on the side.

A few weeks later I saw my way to getting my own back on Sister Meux. The three clinics were about fifteen miles out of the city along the only road leading up-country – Jui was immediately beside the main road, Hastings only another half mile on the opposite side but Grafton was three to four miles away down a dirt road and was the clinic with the poorest attendance rate. In order to save fuel and make the optimal use of the staff we stopped at Jui first, then on to Hastings and after a quick break for lunch went on to Grafton, picking up the nurse from Jui as we headed for home. I normally only went to two out of the three clinics in order to save time and petrol but I left it to Sister to allocate the staff, including myself, as she thought best.

The Grafton clinic was the least popular with all of us, mainly because of the paucity of patients but also because the attitude towards us in the barracks was cool to put it at its best. The small concrete room in which we consulted had a veranda with a bench on which the patients waited. This was invariably covered in goat dung and the room itself was supposed to be scrubbed out each week after we had gone. The so-called Sergeant Major in charge of the barracks was an untidy old man with a jaw half full of rotten teeth. The only time we had ever seen him in uniform was when the President's wife ceremonially opened a Muslim orphanage in the district and he had to make an official appearance.

We would jolt round to the front of the little clinic and confirm that it was in its usual dirty state and then trundle our way through the lines of concrete boxes until we were outside his lordship's house. Then, a long blast on the horn and he would appear half dressed and looking very surprised to see us. He would call to some unseen person in the back of the hut and we would bump our way back down the lines. In due course a small skinny child of seven or eight, bare-footed and wearing only a ragged T-shirt and abbreviated skirt would appear carrying in one hand a bucket a third full of water in which a filthy cloth sloshed about and, in the other, a native broom of tied twigs. This was used to brush the goat droppings onto the earth at the foot of the veranda. Then the child would get down on her hands and knees and wipe the cloth in wide sweeps over the floor. Attempts to encourage the Sergeant Major to arrange for the place to be cleaned before we arrived and to have it done more effectively had proved fruitless and we just accepted the status quo.

On this Tuesday Sister Meux asked me to go to Jui and then Hastings so that I would not be attending Grafton for the second week running. I am sure this was just a mistake on her part and she had forgotten that we had had the same arrangement the week before, but it gave me my opportunity.

"I know why you don't want me to go to Grafton, it's because you've got your eye on the Sergeant Major and you don't want me to see you together!"

The other nurses thought this was a huge joke and laughed until the tears came down their cheeks. The thought of the fastidious Sister Meux associating with that dirty old scallywag was very funny but I was a little apprehensive in case I had gone too far and she did not think it was such a joke. I need not have worried.

"Doctor Wilson, how can you suggest such a thing!" she said with a smile. "You know MY boy friend is the Officer in Charge of Training at Hastings." As we all knew that this personage was a married middle-aged woman, I think we ended up all square.

Hastings was the Police Training Barracks and the single story huts were spread out over a considerable area. The new recruits, both men and women were drilled rigorously, their heads were shaved, more, I gathered, so that they could be quickly identified if they ran away than for the reasons of hygiene. The camp was tidy and well kept and was the only place where I ever saw a live cow, two in fact. These were said to belong to the Commanding Officer to provide him with fresh milk every day. They were Guernseys and looked very well-groomed and healthy. The Commanding Officer lived on the site but also had a house in Freetown where his wife was a teacher in a secondary school. The other permanent members of the training staff also lived on site with their families and these women provided the bulk of our patients. Many came for ante-natal care, some for family planning and a few with gynaecological or infertility problems.

Keturah was particularly good at relating to the women and she would go off 'motivating' while Sister and I saw the patients. One woman, Regina, became very active in promoting contraception, especially the 'chook' (injection of Depo Provera), and came to see us nearly every week, frequently bringing a friend. She was also a source of 'coal' or charcoal. Most of the Marie-Stopes nurses cooked on charcoal. It was not only cheaper to buy it outside the city but, by means of the Land-Rover, we were often able to deliver the dirty hessian sacks at, or near, the recipient's home. The bags were loosely tied and the bulging lumps of charcoal were covered with leaves but this did not prevent a constant leak of black dust escaping, not only from the top but also from the numerous holes in the hessian. We frequently had 'orders' for two or three bags and these plus those wanted by our own team meant that the whole of the back of the vehicle was piled high and Keturah had to balance herself precariously along one of the narrow facing seats.

I took a photograph of Regina carrying the heavy sack of charcoal on her head, the last of five for that day, bare-breasted and with a wide grin on her face. She had had her third injection of depo-provera that morning and was delighted not to be pregnant. The youngest of her five children was now two and a half. She was twenty five and had never had such a long interval free of pregnancy since she was married at sixteen. She felt that five children were sufficient for them to feed and clothe properly but was afraid her husband would insist on having more before very long. Today's injection would protect her for another three months and possibly longer, so for the moment, she was happy.

We arrived one Tuesday at Grafton about 1.30 and as soon as the place had been cleaned up, the equipment carried in from the Land-Rover and the clinic set up, a tall well built man in his fifties came hurrying across the rough ground in front carrying a small child in his arms. His wife was almost running to keep up with him. They had obviously been watching from their house in the lines until we were ready to start.

"Come in, sit down. What is the matter with the pikin?" asked Sister.

"She is my grand-daughter, her name is Alice. She is a refugee from Liberia." He spoke in excellent English. "Her parents put her on a boat in Monrovia to escape the civil war. I don't know what's happened to them but the child got separated somehow from the friends who were supposed to be looking after her and now she is dying from starvation."

Indeed the little girl who, her grandfather said, was twenty one months old, was very small, her limbs like sticks one might use for kindling and her face shrunken so that she looked like a small monkey. Her eyes were enormous and gazed apathetically in front of her with no attempt to look at her surroundings. Even when we had to lift her from his arms to place her in the sling and weigh her, she remained inert.

"Four point five kilos," said Keturah. About nine pounds I translated to myself. I picked up a loose fold of skin from the child's abdomen. When released the tissue only gradually uncreased itself and slowly slid back into the rest of the integument. There appeared to be no subcutaneous fat left and she was obviously seriously dehydrated.

"We got a message that she was on the boat and we only found her this morning."

I remembered hearing of a ship full of refugees who had at first been refused permission to land because Freetown was already inundated with people fleeing from Liberia. By the time it was allowed to dock, many were dead or dying. These grandparents were desperate with anxiety and the picture they presented was made even more poignant as they had bathed and cleaned the tiny mite and dressed her in a spotless pink frock that would have looked lovely on a child going to a party.

"Pa, this pikin is very sick but you can save her. You must give her small, small drinks of water with sugar and salt in it, as we shall tell you. You must try and give her one pint water every two hours, then when she is a little stronger you mix some milk powder with the water, at first small but then stronger."

Sister went on to give them further instructions which the grandfather wrote down after he had tenderly placed the child in his wife's arms.

It was a week before we were back in Grafton and we all nearly cheered when we saw the old couple sitting on the bench outside the clinic awaiting our arrival with little Alice sitting up on her grandfather's lap watching our approach with interest. She was wearing a pretty yellow dress on this occasion and was still too weak to stand unaided on the scales we normally used for toddlers, but her eyes were alert and she pointed to me and wanted to see my glasses which I took off and allowed her to handle. Her weight had gone up by two pounds, some of it no doubt due to rehydration but she was looking like a little girl now and no longer resembled a dying monkey.

When we held our Marie-Stopes Christmas party in Grafton it was almost impossible to recognise the mischievous two year old running about impatiently looking for her coloured paper hat, except that young Alice was wearing quite the most beautiful frock of all the attractively dressed toddlers and the eyes of the loving grandparents who had saved her life watched with pride and joy as she displayed her undoubted skills dancing to the rhythm of the 'tape' with no sign of weakness or disability.

Chapter 4 – November.

Go, Go, Doc. There is the Main Road

ISABELLE, THE PARTIALLY SIGHTED WIFE of a VSO, who taught at the Blind School asked me to talk to the children about simple hygiene and health problems. There were between forty and fifty children resident ranging in age from six to eighteen. They were divided into two groups roughly corresponding to primary and secondary pupils, as age was not a useful guide to their level of education which depended largely on their understanding of English. The children came from all over Sierra-Leone and their tribal languages were distinct. They spoke to each other in Krio but they were taught in English. Most of the older pupils were trilingual and were also learning Braille. The school had only recently acquired two second hand Braille typewriters.

The younger children were shabbily dressed in not very clean shirts and shorts or faded dresses that were missing buttons and belts. Some wore flip-flops but many were bare-footed. Twelve had oozing tropical ulcers on their lower legs, and most had more than one. The sores did not appear to be painful unless touched or knocked accidentally but they were very unsightly and left to themselves would take months to heal. As the children and nearly all the staff were blind, I think few people were even aware that there was such a problem. Many pupils suffered minor ailments, the ubiquitous scabies mite being the primary cause of most of the skin lesions as the children scratched the itchy burrow which then became infected creating an open sore which could rapidly increase in size until some sort of equilibrium with the host's resistance was reached. Coughs and colds were common and most suffered minor attacks of malaria at some time during their stay at school. The older ones tended to complain of headaches and body-aches which they distinguished from bouts of malaria.

I arranged with the Headmaster to call in to the school three times a week on those days when I finished my work early enough and to hold a 'sick parade' regularly. I carried a stock of paracetamol, chloroquine and a few other commonly used drugs which I could dispense on the spot and if other medication was required I could collect it the next day and hand it in on my way home. In the past, any child who felt ill reported to one of the few staff and then had to be escorted to the main clinic by the only seeing person on the site, apart from Isabelle. William had a multitude of multifarious duties and a visit to the clinic could take one or two hours so we tended to see only those children, who, like Fatu, were really sick. I kept a careful record of the supplies I took for the use of the Blind School and refunded the dispensary accordingly.

I consulted the nurses about the best way of tackling the horrible sores on the children's legs. Eusol, an old-fashioned antiseptic lotion seemed to be the favourite but several others were recommended. I had tried them all with varying degrees of success before all the sores were healed. Whatever fluid was applied, a pledglet of gauze had to be soaked in it and the dressing then had to be held in place until my next visit. There were eleven children from six to thirteen in my first ulcer session in the dark little 'surgery'. I started on the eldest first, hoping that Osman would be stoical enough to set a good example to the younger ones. I had a bottle of Eusol and some cotton wool to clean the surrounding skin which was encrusted with dried exudate spilling over the rim of the lesion and running down the boy's leg. As I started to rub the moistened cotton wool gently round the sore I was momentarily horrified to see that the swab had become black. For a split second I thought I had removed the pigment from his skin and then realised that it was, in truth, dirt.

At this time there was no matron or house-mother at the school and nobody appeared to be responsible for supervising the washing arrangements. There was a good supply of cold water from the tap in the yard but what child will wash himself properly if there is no-one supervising the operation? Fortunately Osman made no complaint, in fact he chatted cheerfully while I cleaned him up and then applied the dressing. One or two of the younger children were not so brave and William had to hold them. But he was gentle and the protests were sobs rather than screams. It took me nearly an hour to deal with all the patients but it was time well spent Not only were all the sores healed in time for the annual prize-giving and open day at the end of term but I got to know these children a little better because I was seeing them three times a week.

I had other concerns about the pupils health and asked to speak to the Headmaster. I wanted to know what were the diagnoses concerning their blindness when they came here. Perhaps some of the them would benefit from treatment. I'm not an expert but I have a friend who works at the Kissy Eye Hospital who says she would be glad to help us.

"Well, Doctor Wilson, all the students were examined not long ago by a specialist from Lunsa so you see we are doing our best."

"Of course Headmaster, I know that, but it seems a pity not to make use of my friend's expertise as it's available and will cost nothing. Perhaps I could have a look at the records made by the eye specialist from Lunsa?"

I knew that that was the main ophthalmic hospital, sited about eighty miles from Freetown. The Kissy Eye Hospital was for out-patients only and was mainly staffed by nurses but a consultant came down from Lunsa in January for three months each year to operate and assess the less straightforward cases. I wanted to make sure that these children had each been examined by Hilary before the start of the school holidays so that any who might benefit from surgical treatment would be identified and their parents consulted before the start of the next term in January.

The Head's ability to make his way round the school, and, in particular, his dark and dusty office, without hesitation or stumble made it difficult to remember that he was totally blind but when he opened the cupboard the consequences were all too apparent to those who could see. Both deep shelves were covered with a higgledy-piggledy collection of old brown cardboard folders, randomly tossed one on top of another.

"Can you find the file with the children's medical records for Doctor, Mr Andrews?" he asked in his deep melodious voice.

Mr Andrews was not visually impaired but it took him nearly twenty minutes to locate the right dusty folder. I glanced at it quickly to make sure it was what I wanted. At first I was unsure but then I found several pages at the back headed 'Assessment by Dr Torrah' and the date – May 1989, nearly eighteen months before, with a table listing the children by name, followed by the diagnosis and a final column for any recommended treatment.

"Would it be possible for me to borrow this?" I asked tentatively. "It would be easier for me to study it properly at home."

"Of course, of course." I knew by now that this was his favourite expression. He was always anxious to do all that he could to help.

Now I had the all-clear and could start to make the practical arrangements. I had been invited to tea on Sunday by Hilary and her husband Tom. They were both employed by an Anglican missionary society but worked professionally for different local organisations, she as a specialist nurse at the Eye Hospital and he as a lecturer in theology at the University. They lived in an airy house high on the Fourah Bay campus, two miles up a steep snaking road leading up from the slums of Freetown. Their power supply, like mine by this time, was almost non-existent and their water pressure was minimal but the view was eye-catching and the house was surrounded by tall trees interspersed with scrubby bushes. The danger from snakes was very real and Hilary had twice opened her back door to find a green mamba on the step and spitting cobras in the concrete drainage ditches round the house were nothing to be surprised about. In spite of the difficulties they were a most hospitable couple and frequently had friends and students visiting them at weekends when Hilary was not working. During the hours of daylight we would sit in the breeze and enjoy a cup of tea and a piece of home made cake, boiled in a tin.

She finished work at the Eye Hospital in the early afternoon and I arranged to pick her up on my way back from my Thursday clinic so that we could go to the Blind School when the pupils' studies were finished. The children were assembled in a gloomy dark classroom and were marshalled five at a time on a wooden bench. Hilary examined each one carefully using a powerful torch and her ophthalmoscope, while I recorded her findings.

Unhappily most of the children were totally and irreversibly blind, but not all and a few were suffering pain and discomfort which could possibly be alleviated by the correct treatment. We departed finally about five o'clock after two hours of intensive effort. Some of the younger children had not been very anxious to cooperate at the start of the exercise but in the end they had become convinced that we were not going to hurt them or take them away.

We had an hour of daylight in which to return to my flat and compare our findings with the records made eighteen months before. I was pleased to see that my confidence in Hilary's professional skill had not been misplaced. Her diagnosis of each child's condition correlated almost exactly with that of the previous findings by the eye specialist from Lunsa. He had recommended four pupils for surgery and one who was extremely short-sighted only needed a pair of very strong spectacles to enable her to see almost normally. One of these students had left the Milton Margai more than a year ago but the others were still in school. Nothing had been done to implement the recommendations and, as far as the outcomes were concerned, his visit had been a total waste of time. Five children had joined the school in the last eighteen months and Hilary thought that one of these might have a chance of sight with suitable surgery. I would have to have a session with the Headmaster and make arrangements for the pupils to be taken to the Kissy Eye Hospital for official reassessment and possible surgery.

Friday was always a long day. I left my compound by 7.30am, driving away from Wilkinson Road, climbing up the looping curves of Spur Road, past the British High Commission Compound, past the military hospital (no water and no power for months) and the military barracks, past that relic of the Raj, Hill Station, the ironic reminder of life in Freetown eighty years ago when a working railway carried the British colonials from their airy spacious houses on the hills down into the sweltering heat of the town below. I turned left into Hill Cot Street and saw a schoolgirl standing at the side of the road. I recognised the green uniform of the Annie Walsh Methodist School for Girls which was founded in 1843. It was built in what was then the residential part of the town but which is now embedded in the steaming slums of the East end. My route would take me within 300 yards of the school so I stopped and she quickly got in. Although many think nothing of covering two or three miles on foot, nearly all the school children depend on lifts from private motorists or, if they are unlucky, taxis, to transport them if it is too far to walk. As the weeks went by I built up a regular clientele of schoolgirls – different ones on each day of the week according to my varying schedule. Elizabeth told me she was hoping to go to University to study science but she had exams to pass and two more years at school before she would know whether this was going to be possible. Her English was not at all fluent. I knew this was the language of secondary education and all statutory examinations but, that apart, her problems were only just beginning. The schools had been closed for five months earlier in the year because of a teachers' strike, as the government had been unable to pay them and there was no reason to suppose this would not happen again. Parents not only had to pay fees and buy books and uniforms they had to pay for the use of a desk and chair and, in many cases, give the teacher a 'dash' to ensure that their child received an adequate amount of staff time. Even if, after years of studying, she succeeded in getting a place at Fourah Bay, what chance had she of any true higher education at a university without books, electricity or water?

We drove down Hill Cot Road over the bridge which was the site of the failed coup on the President's life in 1986, into Pademba Road, past the forbidding walls of the jail where six of the conspirators had been executed, and turned right into Circular Road. The traffic was building up but was still fluid. I waved to Hilary as she stood waiting for her pick-up by Brian, employed by the Overseas Development Administration, who gave her a lift to Kissy Eye Hospital every morning. I turned right by the burnt out shell of a past Kingdom Hall of the Seventh Day Adventists and down the steep one-way street. This was cluttered now with school-children, women going to market, small boys with two-foot trays on their heads and men walking unconcernedly down the middle of the street so that it was essential to use the horn repeatedly. At the bottom I said goodbye to Elizabeth and pulled into the abomination of Kissy Road.

Freetown is on a peninsula about thirty miles long and ten wide, connected to the south western edge of Sierra Leone by a narrow neck not more than three miles across. Time was when a passable road ran all round the peninsula from Waterloo on the main land mass, along the fifteen miles to Freetown on the south west corner of the peninsula through the city and along the beautiful Atlantic coast to the south east until, hugging the sea, it reached the end, curved round to the north side and eventually rejoined the main road just short of Wellington.

Now, the only part at which an attempt is made to keep it in repair, is the access to the capital. All traffic has to travel on this one route as the railway to Bo and the hinterland was sold to the Chinese in 1982 and all that remains are the iron girders of the bridges. These span the numerous water courses that fill up in the rainy season carrying the water down to the sea. The road surface approaching the city is quite good until the Port district is reached, signalled by the Up-Gun roundabout at the end of Kissy Road. The wall of the enormous municipal cemetery lies on one side and a street market on the other. Nearer in to the centre, two and three storey buildings with shops open to the street, line the pavements almost without a break. Leaving the town centre behind me the right-hand side was almost unnavigable as a new telephone line had been laid, so I had been told, and the resultant trench had been inadequately filled in. As a consequence the road surface resembled a rift valley which could only be safely traversed by a four-wheel drive vehicle. All other traffic had to trespass onto the left-hand side, dodging precariously through the oncoming trucks, poda-podas (mini-buses) cars and taxis. I knew that by going early there was a good chance of reaching my destination before the worst of the congestion, and so it proved.

I drove into the Ports compound past the dignified but decrepit building of the old Fourah Bay College built in 1865, part of which is used as a minor court of law, the ironwork rusty, and saplings sprouting from the roof. Although it was still only eight o'clock, the old man was

79

already sitting expectantly outside the clinic. He lived by selling empty containers – bottles, jars, cans, cheese boxes etc. Even if there was no lid they were still saleable especially outside the clinic as patients had to provide their own containers for liquid medicines. So many had skin infections that we dispensed gallons of benzoyl-benzoate to treat their scabies and the old man benefited accordingly. Each week I gave him a carrier bag of used Quosh bottles, empty marmalade jars, coke cans if I had been seeing an American friend, Dairylea boxes and anything else I thought he could sell. He emptied them out of the plastic bag and carefully arranged them on the concrete.

Sister Nicol arrived soon after, smiling as she nearly always did, wearing the smart blue uniform dress of the Marie-Stopes staff. She was first identified to me as 'that yaller one' because her skin was lighter than most of her colleagues. We also had a receptionist and sometimes an SECHN (State Enrolled Community Health Nurse). The Port Authority which was German-run, provided a health service for its own employees and their dependants which had a doctor in daily attendance but Marie-Stopes undertook to run an ante-natal, family planning, gynaecological, and venereal disease clinic. We were also allowed to see and treat anyone who lived in the area even if they had no connection with the Port. Our clinic was open every day but I was only there once a week so Sister collected all the patients whom she thought should see a doctor onto a Friday morning.

The first was a police-woman aged twenty eight. She had had a baby ten years before which had been delivered by Caesarian section and had not survived. Subsequently the wound had burst open probably because the suture material was rotten. She had been re-admitted to hospital with a huge gaping wound. Miraculously it had eventually healed by 'granulating up from the bottom' but it was five months before she was allowed home. She was lucky to be alive but she had been left with a solid mass of scar tissue as big as my fist between her umbilicus and public hair line. When I examined her vaginally it was impossible to distinguish the uterus from the rest of the irregular fibrous lump and when I gently moved the mass with my internal finger the skin of her abdomen moved with it. There was obviously no functioning uterus left and conception was completely impossible. She had come to me as a last hope, hearing there was a new woman doctor. She had been attending a private gynaecologist for a year who had been treating her with monthly courses of a very expensive ovulation-inducing drug. I explained to her as carefully as I could that there was no possibility of her ever bearing a child, helping her to feel the monstrous mass of scar tissue in her abdomen and drawing a parallel between the healed but mutilated flesh she could see on the outside and what had happened inside her womb. She understood me without difficulty and naturally was very distressed although I think she had known in her heart of hearts that she would never conceive again. She had consulted many doctors over the years but no-one had attempted to explain to her what the problem was and they had all prescribed treatments and repeated follow-up visits which had taken most of her modest salary. At least she did have her career in the Police and was not reduced to the usual situation of the childless wife at the bottom of the family hierarchy, a slave to all, the last to eat, and the first to be given the most unpleasant jobs to do.

By 11 o'clock nearly all the patients Sister expected had turned up, as well as the usual ante-natal ladies and two men with VD. It was time for me to go on to Kissy clinic which I was not really looking forward to, for several reasons. The first was the journey, the distance was only about three miles, of which the beginning held no problems – along the road towards the neck of the peninsula which still had a good surface and where the traffic was light. However, at the BP garage, past the Shell refinery on the left and the Eye Hospital on the right I had to turn off into Old Kissy Road. The connecting 500 yards was pitted with craters and ruts usually filled with water as this was the rainy season and it was therefore impossible to assess the depth of the holes. Half the 'carriageway' was often obstructed by huge parked trucks, some abandoned, and any vehicles I met were unlikely to yield right of way to my little Ford Fiesta. The T-junction where this feeder road met the Old Road was, in effect, like a village pond which had to be traversed somehow before gaining the dry land, where at least the hazards were visible. The wide road, originally the only route into Freetown was still largely tarmaced but was crossed at fifty yard intervals by horizontal ditches inadequately filled in, the African inverse equivalent of 'sleeping policemen'.

The second reason for my disquiet was the atmosphere in the clinic itself. It was the only place in the Marie-Stopes organisation in which I felt slightly uncomfortable. The two nurses were not impolite but lacked the warmth and spontaneity of the staff at the other clinics. The number of attendances had dropped since these two had been there and I thought this was understandable as their attitude to their clients was rather casual and they often wore their own clothes which was not in accord with Marie-Stopes policy.

There was only one woman waiting with a boy of about seven years old. He hopped in with his mother supporting him, holding his left foot clear of the ground. He had a puncture wound in his heel, probably caused by his bare foot treading on a rusty nail as it was badly infected – the skin tensely swollen and red. He was obviously in great pain and the treatment was to cut it open and let out the pus. He was put on the examination couch, crying pitifully and pulling his foot away every time an attempt was made to touch his heel. The watchman was called in to hold his leg and I then discovered to my horror that the only instrument available to perform this unpleasant procedure was the needle used for giving injections! The nurse set about trying to open up the wound, poking and pricking to let out the thick yellow matter. The child screamed and writhed but there was no alternative.

The pus came out in drops instead of a gush. She tried to squeeze the heel but this was ineffective. Finally the watchman took over and a core of purulent material was extruded and the wound was cleaned with hibitane solution. The boy's agony while all this was being done to him was almost more than I could tolerate and I swore to myself that in future every clinic would be equipped with scalpel blades. One firm incision through the almost dead skin over the top of an abscess is not too painful and it is over in seconds. This child had suffered dreadfully for more than ten minutes, almost entirely because we did not have even basic equipment.

At 2 o'clock I decided to go. There had been no patients for over half an hour and the two nurses left me alone while they stayed in the waiting room, one flirting with the watchman and the other crocheting some object in yellow cotton which never seemed to grow any larger or achieve a definitive shape. I mentioned my difficulties driving along the Old Road, especially the pond at the T-junction. Musu, the watchman told me there was a much better way which he could show me, down one of the back streets. I was aware that he wanted a lift to the town himself but he would not have hesitated to ask for this whichever route I travelled. He was so engagingly enthusiastic it was impossible to refuse.

We crawled out of the police compound into the Old Road but after two or three hundred yards he directed me down an unpaved side-turning. We crept unhappily over the red earth puddles and turned left along an even more uninviting track, clumps of leafy vegetation scraping the underside of the car. After half a mile or so I could see no way forward but Musu was undeterred.

"Go, go, Doc, there is the main road over there." It was true that by stretching my neck I could see the tops of a few trucks moving at some speed but the reason I could not see them properly was because there was a bank at least four feet high between us and the highway. Undismayed he told me there was a ramp further along by which it could be crossed.

By this time I had realised that however good a route this was for a pedestrian, it was inappropriate for a small saloon car. However, there was nowhere to turn, so I crawled on. Sure enough, there WAS a ramp – of a kind! It crossed the earth bank at right-angles at a gradient which I estimated to be 1 in 3, and I was unable to see the other side. I got out and climbed the muddy slope with some difficulty. The top was only about two feet across and the descent down the far side equally precipitous. The whole structure was little more than a yard wider than the car. I backed a little, having decided that I would need considerable acceleration to reach the top. I had visions of getting up, only to be stranded over the summit with neither set of wheels touching the earth. Somehow we scrambled over and slithered down the other side. Ahead lay the dual carriageway that led to Freetown.

The presence of a single-wire fence was not going to deter me at this stage and I told the slightly less exuberant Musu to gather three of the ever present observers of our difficulties and get them to stand on the very loose wire so that it was on the earth and I could drive over it. This they were only too delighted to do, in fact so many came to help that it was difficult to decide to whom I should give a 'dash'. With a now triumphant Musu beside me I reached the tarmac. What neither he nor I had worked out before we started was that we were joining the right hand lane of the dual carriageway which, of course, led out of the city.

I had to drive five miles in the wrong direction before I could make a U-turn and head back to Freetown. Three-quarters of an hour after leaving the clinic I passed the BP garage. It would take at least half an hour to reach my longed for goal; another mile on the good surface, the crawling stops and starts of Kissy Road, the chaos and confusion of the city centre and the final ascent of the pot-holed red laterite track to the British Council.

This is a fine modern building set on a small plateau with wonderful views over Freetown to the harbour and the sea. The edge of the escarpment is shaded by several large trees and the drop protected by a low wall. There was plenty of room to park and when I eventually reached this mecca I heaved myself out of the car and stood for a minute enjoying the light breeze that blew from the ocean. The delights of the British

Council building were many – upstairs it had a good lending library; perhaps women writers, especially those of an independent turn of mind, were over-represented but video and audio cassettes were lent as well as books; there was a large hall where films could be shown or performances staged but it was the ground floor that was my primary objective on Friday afternoons. The ladies loos were clean, sometimes even had paper and usually flushed when required, and water came out of the taps over the hand basins. A visit to them was a pleasant preliminary to the principle pleasures I was anticipating, not a necessity as it would have been in Scotland.

At home my urinary continence depended, especially in the mornings, on ready access to a lavatory, say every two to three hours and at even shorter intervals if I had had something to drink. Not so in Africa. I normally left my flat at seven thirty and had no need to empty my bladder until I got home which was sometimes not until after six. However, the knowledge that the loos were there put the thought into my head and I felt more comfortable if I paid my respects, even if it was only a tablespoonful!

Finally, I walked across to the small cafe, ordered a 7-Up and a toasted cheese sandwich, and sat down to read a ten day old *Guardian* in the bliss of air-conditioning. To me, at that moment, this was as near paradise on earth as I could hope to get.

One Monday afternoon, I recognised a young woman waiting on one of the benches in the entrance to the blind school. Unfortunately I could not remember her name but it did not matter as she recognised my voice and cheerfully greeted me.

"Hello, Doctor Wilson, you see me and my pikin at the clinic." She nursed a tiny infant who looked severely malnourished. The child was eleven months old but weighed less than ten pounds. She was one of twins, born prematurely and her sister had died within a month of birth. It was not surprising as the seventeen year old mother was totally blind and was herself an orphan dependent on the erratic and unskilled help of neighbours to feed and care for herself and her baby. As long as the child was fully breast-fed and the young mother's milk supply was adequate the child had survived but she had never made up for her low birth weight and now that she required supplementary food, which her sightless mother could not prepare for her, she was losing ground rapidly.

They had been at the nutrition clinic and Mamie had been given a supply of high protein powder to add to the baby's feeds. The real problem was that there was no older woman who would act as a 'stand-in mother' on a day to day basis. Mamie came every week to the clinic but the baby hardly gained an ounce and in the middle of the third week she brought the child to see the doctor as she could tell that the baby was very ill. The little scrap had pneumonia and, in spite of all we could do, was dead in twenty four hours.

The young mother seemed to take her loss philosophically but I would often see her sitting on the bench in the entrance with such a sad, resigned expression on her face that I longed to comfort her. All I could do was to stop and talk to her a little of the doings of the day and her face would become animated and smiling. She knew the sound of my car engine and would be standing to greet me before I was out of the driver's seat. After I held my 'surgery' with the children and was on my way out I would see her waiting, as I had seen her many times when her baby was alive, only now she was alone.

One Friday evening in late November I was locking the second padlock on my door when I felt a sudden sting in my left eye. I thought a bit of grit had blown in with the evening breeze and tried the old trick of pulling my upper lid over the lower to try and dislodge it or wash it out with the subsequent lachrymation. This was not successful so I wasted no more time in getting into the Fiesta and driving to Leona's flat at the Bintumani. We had arranged to go for a meal together at Roots, one of the local restaurants, after enriching our spirits by watching the sunset from her balcony while enjoying a 'Star'.

"I wonder if you'd mind looking in my eye? I think I've got a bit of grit in it."

Leona separated my lids with her fingers and examined it carefully.

"No, I can't see anything there, but it's kinda red."

It was also beginning to be quite painful but there was nothing more I could do about it at that moment, so we finished our beer and both getting into my car, went off to Roots. This was a delightful establishment with tables set out on terraces that overlooked the little inlet between Aberdeen Village on its wooded knoll and the Cape Sierra mini-peninsula. There was a pleasant breeze from the sea and the tables on the upper terrace were protected from the unpredictable tropical downpours by a palm thatched roof, open at the sides so that there was no obstruction to wind or view.

The food was delicious and was always served by one of the proprietor's many nubile wives. He was a man in his forties who had lived for many years in the United States but had returned to his native Sierra-Leone and set up in the restaurant business. He needed a source of reliable labour both to help him in the kitchen and to wait on the customers. He solved the problem by marriage to an increasing number of very attractive young women. I think he had six at this time, having recently advertised for an additional two as one of the earlier contingent was very pregnant and another had a full time job looking after the several small children he had already fathered.

There was no shortage of applicants. He was a good husband and father and also had a well-founded reputation for being a good business man. Any wife of his would be assured of a full belly and comfortable living in exchange for learning the mysteries of how to be the perfect waitress and improving her English. This evening we were served by a very attractive young woman who spoke good English with a slight American accent and whose bare feet were almost silent as she glided between the tables. Leona and I both chose sea-food platters and finished off the meal with ice-cream, a luxury we did not often have the opportunity of enjoying. By the time I was driving back to the hotel I could no longer see clearly out of my left eye and the right was beginning to feel gritty. Leona got out and said goodnight with several expressions of anxiety about the state of my eye which was obviously affected by something more virulent than a bit of grit.

As soon as I was safely locked up inside my flat I opened my so-far-unused medical kit I had brought out with me. I was fairly certain I was suffering from a very severe attack of acute conjunctivitis which was known locally as 'Apollo Eye'. I had seen two or three cases in the clinic but not recently, and the source of my present affliction remained a mystery. By the light of my torch I found the little tube of tetracycline eye ointment and applied an extruded thread along both my lower lids. Fortunately the next day was Saturday and it was not my turn to do the morning shift at Collegiate School Road. I could not see at all out of my left eye and had restricted vision in the right because both were surrounded by gross peri-orbital oedema. The soft tissue swelling of upper and lower lids had even spread across the bridge of my nose so that my face looked a grotesque mask. It was with great difficulty that I managed to apply the eye ointment to the conjunctiva and had to repeat the operation every four hours.

I could not read or drive, indeed it would have been very antisocial to expose any of my friends to the possibility of infection and I was worried in case Leona might have acquired it in spite of her scrupulous hand-washing both before and after she had looked for the invisible 'foreign body'. That Saturday was a very long day but the power came on totally unexpectedly for three hours in the afternoon so my discomfort was alleviated by the air-conditioner during the sweatiest part of the day. Next morning there was a slight improvement although it took a little while to realise this as both eyes were completely gummed up with gunge and I had to feel my way to the wash-basin and the never failing gush of nearly cold water from the tap so that I could slunge off the accretions of the night. As the day wore on I realised that I could see out of both eyes although neither opened fully, and they were no longer really painful although still very uncomfortable.

Monday dawned and I was able to go to work. The nurses all exclaimed in horror when they saw me.

"You sure got Apollo, Doctor Wilson. Don't you come too near me," said Lauretta, only half joking.

At the end of the clinic I decided to go to a pharmacy and try to get some antibiotic eye drops, rather than continue using the ointment which did appear to be working, but only slowly. I drove in towards the town and drew up at a chemists opposite the small hospital that was run by the Sheffield trained surgeon who was looking after Fatu from the Blind School.

I went in to the rather dark long narrow shop with a counter at the end. There was no nonsense about needing a prescription the only difficulty was whether they had any chloromycetin eye drops in stock.

"You're in luck, Doctor, I've just this one bottle left."

"How much is that?" I asked the man.

"Fifteen hundred leones," he said. Translated into £sd this was about £5 at the current rate of exchange and might not have been considered exorbitant by Western standards but I had been in Freetown long enough to know that a local would have been charged a third of that price. I said nothing and walked out with the tiny vial inside its rather grubby cardboard container. As soon as I reached home I applied a drop of the precious liquid into each eye but I did notice that round the neck of the minute bottle there was a slightly yellow encrustation. I repeated the application twice more before I went to bed but in the morning my eyes were once more closed with exudate although the swelling was no worse. I returned to my slow but genuine ointment and by the end of the week I was cured. As far as I know, no-one else caught the infection.

When my visual acuity had returned to normal I examined my expensive purchase with great interest. The little bottle was made of brown glass, as was normal to protect the contents from the light, but the dropper, integrated into the stopper, was of clear glass and I drew up some of the liquid into the barrel. It was colourless. Chloromycetin is yellow, as its name suggests and I have no doubt the active ingredients had been used long before, judging by the unclean outer cardboard; the empty vial had been refilled from the tap but not without leaving some tell-tale traces of the original contents round its neck.

That attack of conjunctivitis was the only infection of any kind from which I suffered during the time I was in West Africa.

Sunday, but far from a day of rest as far as I was concerned. Sylvia picked me up at 9am to take me with her to the fortieth anniversary of the Christchurch, Pademba Road, Mother's Union. It was as well I did not know, when I set out, how long it would be before I returned! The church is a large one built on exactly the same plan as a contemporary building in Edwardian England – a very wide nave, the pews facing forward, then two banks of chairs facing each other across the aisle for the VIPs, before the steps up to the chancel. There was a very dusty organ as well as a piano. The first four or five rows in the nave were filled with the serried ranks of the members of the Mother's Union wearing white with blue sashes and white hats with blue bands round the crown. I noticed that in one respect at least, this Mother's Union did not differ from its English parent body as I remembered it – the average age of the ladies was well over forty, in fact most seemed nearer sixty which reinforced my belief that it should be renamed the Grandmother's Union.

To my dismay Sylvia firmly led me to the VIP seats. I was the only European in the church which, after the usual passage of considerable time invariably associated with any African ceremony, was filled with an enthusiastic congregation of men, women and children. The service was extremely long. After about three-quarters of an hour the Bishop of Bo went into the pulpit to preach. I thought this heralded the beginning of the end but it was only the end of the beginning. After a few introductory words which I did not hear properly he moved from English into Krio. I followed most of the story which concerned the devoted love of a mother monkey and lasted twenty minutes. I relaxed as he switched into English once more, expecting the blessing, only to hear him say.

"Now we have spoken to the children we will turn to the sermon proper." This lasted a further thirty five minutes. There were a lot of hymns, many with six or eight verses. In the course of the service there were no less than four processions of the congregation up to the altar and back (twice bearing financial offerings), once for the individual blessing of every past, present and, it appeared to me, potential future member of Christchurch, Pademba Road Mother's Union. The final approach up the chancel was a delightful procession of all the children who were each given a flower or small posy from two huge bouquets on either side of the altar, to take back to their mothers. I was amazed to see how many 'pikins' of all ages emerged from the seats, some so small they were carried by a parent, and yet there had hardly been a cry and certainly no unruly shouts or noise for over four hours!

When the first collection was made it was preceded by an exhortation from the Mother's Union President for all to give generously and in particular for anyone with dollars or sterling notes to search their hearts, and their pockets. All the time she was speaking she fixed me with an unwavering stare from the front row of the facing seats which was intended to be observed by all of the congregation within visual range. I felt very uncomfortable. I had not brought any foreign currency with me to church and in any case I had barely enough at home to cover what was required when leaving the country. Even if I had had more I did not feel like giving to this particular section of the community who were all well fed, judging by the girth of most of those present, and who were largely drawn from the ranks of the professional middle class. However, I could not embarrass Sylvia by letting my thoughts appear openly so I wrote 'IOU $10 and will let you have it later' and put this into the envelope provided. I then crossed the aisle in the wake of the official collectors and gave it to my friend of the beady eye.

The large numbers of people who were required to perambulate up the aisle and back again meant that each processional hymn had to be sung several times all the way through as there appeared to be a taboo on changing tunes in mid-march. As a result we sang *Onward Christian Soldiers* six times, all eight verses, two of which I had never heard before.

At 1.20 the service was finally over, although most people were going down to the undercroft for some form of holy bun fight. I was very relieved when Sylvia said she had had enough and asked me if I felt the same. We crept out feeling slightly guilty but knowing we had done nearly all that was required of us, as long as I did not forget to honour my IOU!

On a subsequent Sunday afternoon I drove up to the Shepherds knowing I would receive a welcome and an invitation to stay for a meal and watch a video afterwards. It was one of the weekends when their steward had gone up-line to Port Loko to see his family, so Kelly was doing the cooking.

"I wonder if Desmond will be coming?" she said through the open kitchen door.

"He's usually here by now on a Sunday" said Ken.

"Who's Desmond?" I asked.

"Oh, haven't you met him yet?" Ken replied. "He's a White Father with a parish about twenty miles out of town on the main road up country. He's on his own and feels pretty lonely at times. We keep a bed for him for whenever he feels like it and he usually turns up on Sundays after he's said mass."

"He was in a terrible road accident in Italy. I think it was when he was training to be a priest. Anyway he had a very severe head injury and was unconscious for weeks. Nobody thought he would survive let alone recover completely. He still gets dreadful headaches and they are worse when he is under stress, and that must be most of the time, living as he does." Kelly's compassion was as usual, translated into a very practical form, the comforts of civilisation, good food and friendly undemanding company for any friend who needed it.

I learnt later that when they were on leave, they lent their comfortable, airy house and the steward and house-girl with it, to some of the Catholic sisters who worked all the year round in mission hospitals and schools a hard day's journey or more from Freetown. The week or two the nuns spent in the Shepherds' house was their only holiday and it was very much appreciated.

They themselves had no personal connection with the Catholic church, indeed I am sure they were brought up in a strong Yorkshire non-conformist tradition even if they no longer attended chapel. Ken carried loyalty to his county into his everyday diet and whatever dish we had for dinner, steak, fish pie or macaroni cheese, Ken always had Yorkshire pudding served with it. Kelly had trained the African cook·so well that I think the best Yorkshire I have tasted was made by their Mende steward.

As we were about to sit down to lamb chops (imported through an American freezer company), potatoes (local), carrots (local), peas (frozen from local supermarket) and of course, Yorkshire pudding, Father Desmond O'Ryan arrived. He was a tall, dark, quiet, good-looking man, probably in his early thirties, but he looked exhausted and very hot and sweaty. Brief introductions were made and then he excused himself to have a shower and change his clothes. We did not wait for him but Kelly kept his dinner hot and when he returned he looked ten years younger and was able to tuck in to his substantial meal with gusto. Before we settled down to the serious business of watching an American 'B' movie on the video there was plenty of time for conversation and he invited me to visit him in his parish one Saturday. Kelly said she would be delighted to provide transport and be my guide as I had so little petrol that I had to husband every ounce and would certainly not have been able to make a round trip of fifty miles or so using what was, in effect, Marie-Stopes fuel. I was pleased that Kelly was to be included and we arranged to fix a date when I had no Saturday morning clinic.

It was several weeks before we found a mutually convenient day. Kelly picked me up and we drove out to Waterloo to see Desmond's parish and have lunch with him. Kelly had been before and was able to find his house, opposite the small dilapidated church, without difficulty, but there was no sign of Father O'Ryan or his truck. His steward said he had gone to the clinic as an old man had been taken ill and had been carried there by his son. He offered to show us the way and we bumped back onto the surfaced road and after a further mile or so we saw it set back in a clearing in the bush. Desmond came to meet us,

"I'm afraid we're all too late, the patient has been taken home again by his family."

"Why didn't we meet him as we were coming here?" asked Kelly.

"His son is carrying him on his back and it's nearly two miles by road but there is a track through the bush which cuts off a big corner. Still, he's probably not reached home yet so you might as well see the clinic while you're here."

We were introduced to the Dispenser, employed by the government to run the daily out-patient facility and dispense the drugs he thought appropriate. The short middle-aged man was unpleasantly obsequious and eager to demonstrate his importance. He showed us the usual bottles of vitamins, chloroquine, ampicillin and anti-worm pills and asked the only customer there to show us what he had bought. Eight separate little packets were produced, much to the satisfaction of the dispenser who obviously believed variety was the stuff of life. As each medicament meant money in his pocket he was right from his own point of view. Father O'Ryan said his wages had not been paid for four months and it was therefore entirely reasonable that he should make what income he could from the sale of drugs. We were then taken round the rest of the maternity unit. The labour ward contained four iron bedsteads, without mattresses and an enamel bucket, all covered in dust and debris. When we asked if

91

we could go inside, the key to the padlock on the door could not be found. The two midwives were stretched out on benches in the shade enjoying a quiet snooze and not expecting to be discovered by their boss and three European visitors.

"How many women come to the hospital to be delivered?" I asked the man, in as innocent a tone as I could muster. His answer confirmed my impression that he was extremely stupid (or, of course, that he thought we were).

"We have at least five or six deliveries each week, it's very popular to have a baby in the hospital in Wellington." He then decided he had done his duty by us and went back to his office.

Once he was out of sight I turned to the two women who were by then sitting up looking rather sheepish.

"How long is it since you last had a baby delivered here?"

"I think perhaps two-three weeks," which being translated meant 'not within living memory.' "The women rather have their babies at home with the TBA." I knew this was true and was one of the reasons why the maternal mortality rate was so appallingly high in Sierra-Leone but I did not think delivery in this dirty unprepared maternity unit by one of these pleasant but indolent ladies would have given mother or child a much better chance of survival than the traditional methods. The key to improving the survival of mothers and babies lay in proper training for the TBAs who were trusted and respected by the women in their communities.

Meanwhile Father O'Ryan was becoming a little impatient with all this 'women's talk' and was anxious to get me back to see the sick old man. Kelly drove the car after his truck back to the village and we drew up in front of a small house with corrugated iron roof and cement walls. The door was open and led straight into the front room where the sick man lay on a narrow bed in the corner. At first I could not see him as it was very dark after the brilliant sun outside. The room was no more than eight by ten and all I could see were innumerable people, milling about and talking amongst themselves.

"Ask everyone to go out of the room except his son," I said to Desmond. It was a measure of his authority in the community that the room was cleared with little delay and no fuss and I was able to see the patient lying on his palette in the corner. He was obviously very ill, with rapid respirations and a high fever. The old man was very thin and coughed painfully as I knelt on the floor beside him.

"How long has he been ill?"

"Four-five days; he believes he is going to die," Desmond translated the middle-aged son's reply. The sick man was supported against his son's chest where the latter sat uncomfortably on the top end of the bed. I took my stethoscope out of my brief case which doubled as my handbag. I suspected pneumonia and listened carefully to his chest and watched the working of the alae nasi dilating his nostrils with each laboured intake of breath.

"Lean him forward, would you please, so that I can listen to his back."

There, below his shoulder blades on both sides I heard the crepitations in the lungs which signified the underlying inflammatory process and in one area another physical sign I had not heard for nearly thirty years, which is almost diagnostic of acute lobar pneumonia, the sound of 'bronchial breathing' associated with consolidation of the lung. Vomiting had exacerbated the dehydration of the fever and his skin could be pinched up in dry folds which only sluggishly resumed its normal contours when released.

"Show me the medicine you got from the dispensary this morning."

Seven different dirty little packets of paper were produced, one of which did contain twelve ampicillin capsules. I could tell from their colour that each contained 250 milligrams and in such a severe infection a dose of one gram, ie, four capsules, every six hours for at least the first forty-eight hours was needed. After that, if the patient was improving, the dose might be reduced to two. Ideally he should have had an injection of penicillin but I had none with me and, even if we managed to get some to Father O'Ryan, there was no-one to give it to him. The situation was further complicated as the old man had been vomiting and it seemed likely that even if he managed to swallow all four capsules at once, he might lose the lot five minutes later. I decided on a compromise.

"Give him a drink of clean water with a pinch of salt and four lumps of sugar in it. Give him small, small sips, say up to half a cup. If he is not sick, wait a little, if he does not vomit, give him more of the special water and two of the capsules. We will come back later to see how he is."

Father O'Ryan translated this into Krio and we went back to his presbytery for lunch. I had been very impressed with the loving care which the old man's family, especially his son, had shown and Desmond said this was very typical of how his parishioners treated the elderly members of their community. We had a tasty lunch of pasta in some local sauce and I was then asked to see two more patients in the priest's own household. His steward/cook had a nasty infected finger which needed incising.

"It's a pity I haven't got a scalpel" I said, "because I could open it now and save him a lot of pain. It may take days to burst itself and will then take some time to heal."

"YOU may not have a knife, but I have," said the resourceful Desmond. He went off and I expected him to come back with a Swiss army knife or its equivalent. To my surprise he produced a proper surgeon's scalpel with detachable blade. We boiled it on the paraffin stove for ten minutes to be on the safe side and then I had no difficulty in opening the lesion and letting out the pus. The tense skin alongside the nail was dead and the incision was almost painless but the immediate relief once the tension was gone wreathed Salim's face in smiles and the discomfort associated with cleaning up the wound and applying a clean dressing was virtually unnoticed.

"There's someone else I'd like you to see," said Father O'Ryan. "It's the girl who does my garden. She says she hasn't felt well recently but she swears it's not malaria." He called out of the open door, "Mary, come and see the lady doctor I told you about." Mary had obviously been anticipating the summons and slipped shyly in. She was a slight, pretty girl and did not look ill.

"What age are you?"

"Fifteen years, please Doctor."

"What the matter?"

"De belly dey ache. I not eat."

"How much time this?"

"Two three week."

"You see your monthlies?"

"No monthly," she lifted one finger and then two. I had a shrewd idea of the diagnosis but an examination would clinch it.

"I suppose you haven't a pair of surgical gloves in your treasure trove?" I asked Desmond.

"Well, I have now," he replied in triumph and duly brought me an unused pair of thin rubber gloves.

"I'll just check this lassie. Would you mind if we used your bed as an examination couch? I'll need a small towel and a bowl of water with a bit of soap."

"No problem," said he.

"I check the belly inside," I explained to the girl who did not seem to be at all alarmed at the idea. Sure enough, she was no virgin and was about eight weeks pregnant. I am sure she knew this already but had been afraid to tell the priest because she was not married and she knew the Catholic Church regarded premarital intercourse as a sin. She should have had more faith in Father O'Ryan's compassion.

"I should have thought of that possibility myself," he said. Mary was delighted to know for certain she was going to have a baby and I left it to her and her understanding confessor to work out what she was going to tell her family.

Then we went back to see whether the old man had managed to keep down his capsules. He had, so I gave further instructions and made some complicated arrangements to get some more capsules of double strength back to Father O'Ryan. I am glad to say that the patient did not die although his hold on life was precarious for the next two days. I saw him sitting on a chair in the shade outside his house two weeks later. He was weak but the pneumonia had cleared. I gave him some iron and multi-vitamin tablets as he was certainly anaemic and he had eaten very little when he was ill. Desmond told me a month later that he had fully recovered and said he was stronger than before he was ill.

The themes of the Annual General Meeting of the Sierra-Leone Medical and Dental Association in 1990 were family planning and geriatrics. Who thought of this unlikely twinning between the beginning (or preferable NOT beginning) of life and its ending I do not know but I suspect the outgoing president of the SLMDA. He was a physician of considerable stature (metaphorically speaking, he was, in fact, slim and only of medium height) and foresight; I think he believed that contraception needed to be higher on his colleagues' medical agenda if his country's economic and social problems were ever going to be ameliorated. I have no idea if this was the case but it gave the Marie-Stopes Society an opportunity to appear on the programme. Sylvia submitted my name and the title of the paper, *Twenty years experience with Depo-Provera*.

There was a great deal of active propaganda against the use of this very effective injectable contraceptive emanating from the medical profession which, naturally, affected the attitudes of nurses. As a result it was very under-used. When I started working in the Marie-Stopes clinics I found that it was only being prescribed for women over thirty-five who had a least three children. The doctors' views were the result of lack of knowledge and prejudice. The United States at that time had not licensed this product for general use, not on scientific grounds as it had been endorsed by the official medical experts, but by lay pressure exerted by an alliance of feminists and black power. The former proclaiming that it was being used by male doctors to control women and the latter screaming 'genocide' as it was (incorrectly) said to cause permanent infertility. Personally I have always wondered whether much of this very effective protest was not funded in some way by pharmaceutical companies whose contraceptive eggs lay in the oral or intra-uterine basket.

I was therefore delighted to be able to address the Sierra-Leonian medical establishment on this subject to try and dispel some of the myths, but there were a great many preliminaries to be got through before 10am on Thursday morning. The meeting opened officially on Wednesday with a formal ceremony in the City Hall. Any medically qualified person who was, or who aspired to be, anybody, had to be there. Protocol ruled the morning, there were over twenty personages, almost all men, on the dais and as each rose up to say his piece he addressed his fellows on the platform individually by name and status before coming to the substance of his remarks. Sometimes the laudatory comments extended to colleagues in the audience or even in the graveyard so that the proceedings were somewhat lengthy and I had plenty of time to look around.

On the wall behind the platform were two enormous portraits, one immediately recognisable as our revered and honoured President Mohmoh. The other was of an inscrutable oriental cast of countenance, but definitely not that of Chairman Mao. I subsequently discovered that this was the President of Korea, which Korea my informant did not know, in fact he was surprised to learn that there was more than one. The Koreans had generously paid for the building and fitting out of the handsome edifice in which we were sitting.

Africans love oratory and each made the most of his opportunity to hold forth before an audience of his peers. Many were the elder statesmen of their profession and each had an excellent command of the English language based on matriculation Shakespeare and the authorised version of the Bible. The content, however, did tend to be repetitious and my boredom threshold is not high. Eventually we were released, due to reassemble after lunch at the nearby Connaught Hospital at 2pm.

At ten to two I locked the car and went into the X-ray department above which, I had been told, the rest of the meetings were to be held. There were no patients in the waiting area which was not surprising as the Connaught had neither X-ray film nor power. A lackadaisical custodian directed me upstairs to the fourth floor which, of course, was empty, although one of the rooms was set out like a school-room with about four dozen hard chairs arranged in rows facing a long raised desk.

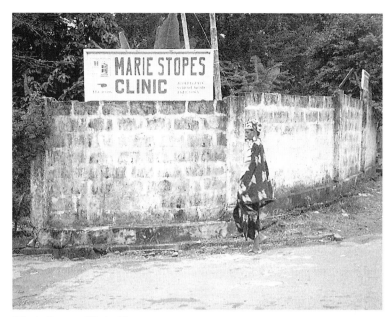

Marie Stopes Clinic, Freetown.

Immunisation campaign. A wrist bangle for every injection.

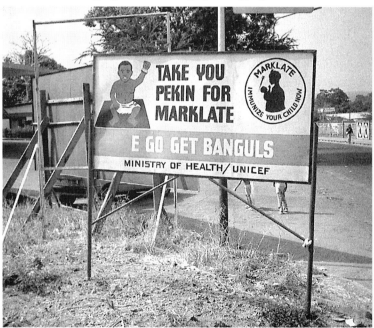

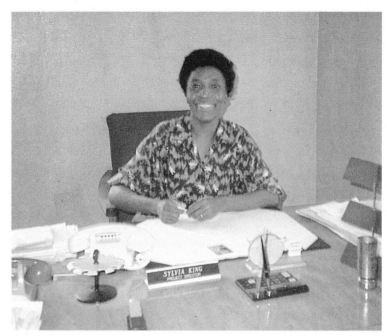

Sylvia Wachuku-King, my boss.

Oranges were cheap and plentiful.

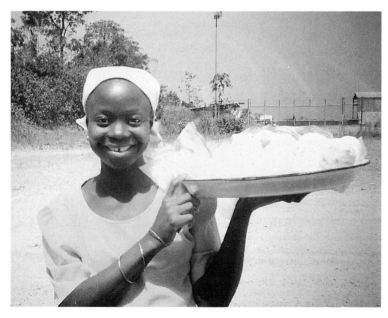

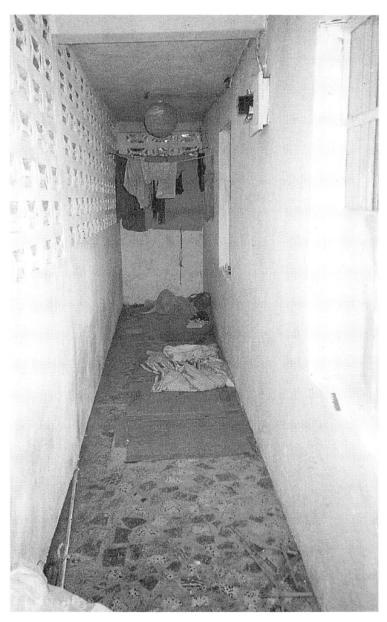

James's (age 16) bedroom, sitting room etc.
The windows looked into my house.

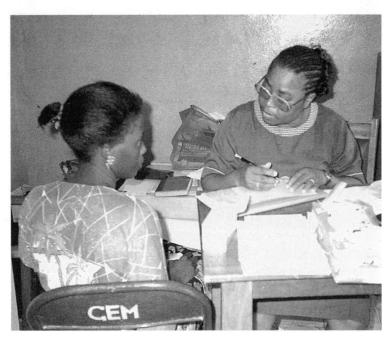

Sister Cline educates a patient about family planning.

Work continues.

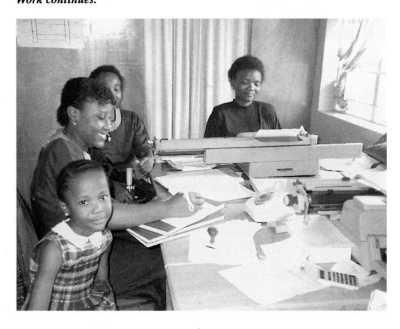

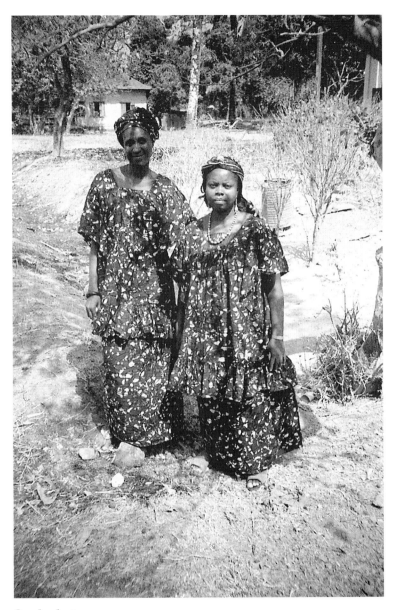

Sunday best.

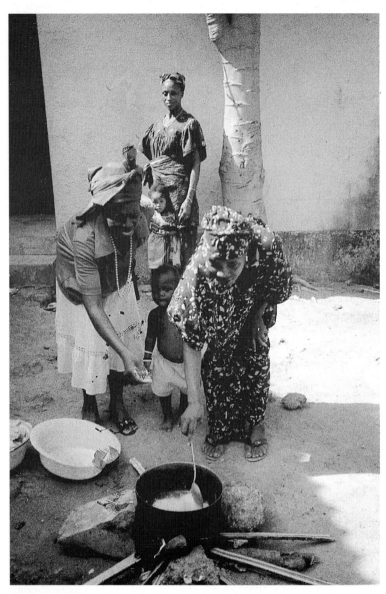

Christmas, 1990.
Family Planning patients start cooking for the party.

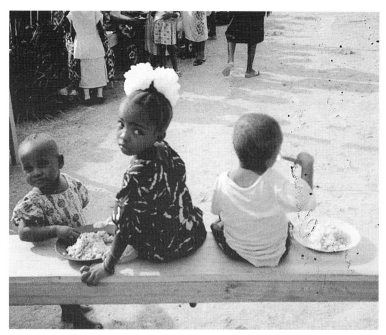

Christmas, 1990 – a good time had by all

The big canoe, Moa.

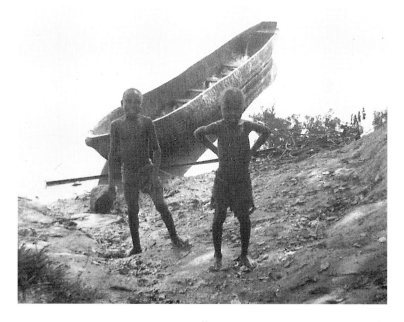

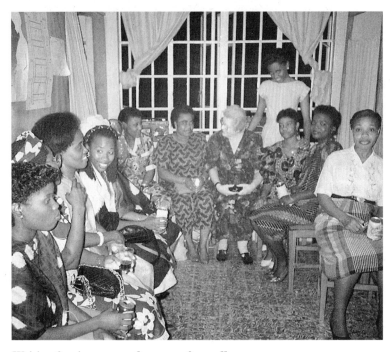

Waiting for sixteen speeches at my farewell party.

By 2.30pm several seats were taken and by 3 o'clock the room was nearly full and the afternoon programme began. Most of the presentations were not very good and some would only have merited a 'D' in the GCSE examination. They were not helped by the absence of any visual aids. It became increasingly hot and sweaty but with the windows open the noises from the street became so intrusive that the lecturers were hard pressed to be heard. After an hour or so it was decided to try and start the fan which was free-standing near the windows. This entailed connecting it to a generator on one of the floors below. The cable was brought through the window and the two naked leads were pushed into the socket of the adaptor attached to the fan. There were a great many sparks and, to me, alarming noises, but the young man manipulating the live wires seemed totally unconcerned and sure enough the fan started to turn. The atmosphere certainly improved and it became much easier to stay awake. The presenter of the final paper had some acetates for use with an overhead projector. This provided a further opportunity for the 'electrician' to demonstrate his skills as there was, of course, no plug on the projector lead and a further alarming firework display was needed before the bulb lit up and the graphs and diagrams could be demonstrated. The wretched lecturer was soon desperately struggling to hold down his flimsy films to prevent them being blown off the machine by the gale created by the fan which was only three feet away and which the shortness of the leads precluded from being moved. In view of these difficulties and because it was the last talk, the fan was turned off. At first it seemed as though his problems were over but no sooner had the transparencies stopped blowing away in the wind than they started to curl up with the heat from the underlying lamp. This proved an insuperable difficulty and in the end the poor man had to abandon all attempts to use them.

I was giving the third paper the next morning and how glad I was that I had had a demonstration of the hazards that lay ahead. I had spent the previous Sunday morning preparing my talk and had made about ten transparencies to illustrate it. I had brought blank acetates, felt tip pens, ruler and pencil with me from the UK. I had also been to the two stationery outlets in the town that I knew of but neither had any idea of what I was talking about. That evening I had to devise a mechanism that would stop my acetates from flying away or curling up when I should be concentrating on what I was saying and not being distracted by mobile transparencies. I also had with me a thick cardboard chart displaying the complex inter-relations of the numerous hormones involved in the reproductive cycle of human females. It was far too complicated for practical use and I had no hesitation in sacrificing it to a more useful purpose. Using the ruler and a Stanley knife (also brought from home) I cut the cardboard into inch wide strips and glued them along the sides and across the top and bottom of each acetate. The result was a firm frame which made them easy to handle and which was sturdy enough to stop them blowing away. It took me nearly two hours to do the job properly by the light of two candles and the need to prevent my sweaty forearm from touching the text, which was hand printed with soluble colours which ran or smudged if any moisture came near them.

I arrived at the lecture room next day at 9 o'clock as directed on the programme. Needless to say, I was the first by forty minutes but the Chairman for the morning session then arrived and I was able to ask him to ensure that the fan and the projector would both be in working order by the time my turn arrived. He then said, "Doctor Baker wants to tell us something about vasectomy. I was going to let him speak for ten minutes or so before your paper."

We were obviously going to be running at least an hour late as it was, and I knew that very few speakers are able to confine themselves to talking for such a relatively short time.

"Would it be possible to put him in after me instead of before?" I asked tentatively. "You see, I've prepared my talk pretty carefully and I can't really cut it short without leaving out some important material." Rather reluctantly he agreed, more because of his innate good manners than because he thought my presentation was worth preserving intact.

Eventually the session started, the hiccups of the previous day were not repeated and, in any case it is not nearly so warm in the morning as it is after noon. The audience was almost entirely male and there were no Europeans amongst the fifty or so doctors present. They were attentive and asked quite a lot of questions at the end which is always a good sign, although I fear I probably did not convince many of them to change their prescribing habits. One asked, "Why did you say that the United States is a poor example for us to follow as far as contraception is concerned?"

"Because they have far less freedom of choice about methods than most other countries in favour of family planning, no I.U.D.s, no injectables, prescribing the pill surrounded by so many regulations that even literate women are deterred and those who become pregnant as a result of using less effective methods risking a bomb in the clinic if they seek an abortion."

I did see several heads nodding in agreement but by then my time was up and the elderly gynaecologist who was the vasectomy expert took over. It was soon apparent that he knew very little about the subject, fortunately too little to spin it out for more than a quarter of an hour. At the end he was asked, "How long after the operation does it become effective."

"Oh, about three or four days."

I felt it was important to set the record straight if I could do so tactfully. I caught the Chairman's eye and he nodded agreement to my making a comment.

"I'm sure that's right for Sierra-Leone but it takes between eighteen and twenty-four ejaculations to clear the sperm from the system." Pause, "In Europe that would take three to four months!"

This brought the house down. The audience laughed as only Africans can laugh even if they are the medical establishment. I think this interjection coming from a white-haired Englishwoman to that virtually all-male assembly made it all the funnier. I certainly got some friendly and good-humoured banter from several of them over the lunch break.

There was an illuminating postscript to the vasectomy talk. The speaker before me was also a woman who had given an excellent presentation on the broader aspects of family planning. She and I were sitting side by side on the 'platform' until the end of the morning session.

"I wonder how many men in the audience would consider having the operation?" I whispered to her. She was a lady of spirit and when the laughter had subsided she asked those who would consider having a vasectomy to raise their hands. Four arms were lifted rather hesitantly. I asked each in turn for their comments.

"I might think about it when I reach the age of seventy."

"Possibly when my youngest wife is past the menopause."

"After my sixth child reaches school age but only if I'm paid half a million leones."

"It's just a joke."

I enjoyed meeting some of my Sierra-Leonian colleagues and putting faces to people who had only been names and professional addresses to me until then. I stood next to the legendary Sister Hilary, a surgeon of international repute who had revolutionised medical and nursing standards in her up-country hospital. She invited me to visit her there and it is one of my on-going regrets that I never managed to do so. The third day was devoted to geriatrics which I felt was not very relevant to most of my work in Freetown. The expectation of life at birth for a male child was forty one years in 1990 and I fear it will be a long time before there is sufficient work for more than one or two geriatric specialists in Sierra-Leone.

Chapter 5 – December
Tell me where I can buy a stamp

DECEMBER, PLENTY TO LOOK FORWARD
to but not much to ease the practical difficulties of my everyday life over
the next two weeks. We had had no power for over a fortnight, not even
in the evening or during the day at weekends. This meant, of course, no
air-conditioning or light but also no fridge. I was still trying to get the
paraffin cooker to work – it took an hour to boil half a kettle of water –
preparing an evening meal had ceased to be a problem as long as I
remembered to buy bread from one of the street vendors in the morning
before they sold out. Fula bread is the best and is a reasonable
accompaniment to a tin of sardines in tomato sauce, half a dozen marble
sized tomatoes and a fresh, sweet, but very pippy orange to follow, washed
down with a warm bottle of 'Star'. I had bought half a dozen eggs the
week before in a moment of mistaken optimism and had only eaten two,
hard boiled at the clinic in the brief hour that the generator was on, but
the remainder had grown beards on their shells. The local version of
margarine was still just edible but I had had to throw out my much
cherished butter.

I ate my supper by candle-light as it was nearly 7 o'clock and already
dark in the flat. It really needed two candles to give enough light to read
by but two candles were so hot, especially when the windows were tightly
closed against mosquitoes. I decided to go outside and read by the light
of the neon-strip lighting which was fixed all round the house to
illuminate the compound to deter thieves and make it easier for the
watchman to detect any nefarious persons. My landlord ran two powerful
generators, one of which was on the veranda directly above my head.
They were extremely noisy and when both machines were in use even
the walls vibrated. I carried an upright 'dining chair' out onto the step,
as the arm chair was too wide and heavy for me to manipulate through
the double doorway. I covered myself with mosquito repellent and
enjoyed an hours read of *The Zim-Zim Road* which Leona had lent me.

By 8.00 my back was screaming for a more relaxed position and I retreated inside and lay on the bed. I struggled with the candles for another forty minutes and then gave up. Fortunately I still had several unheard audio tapes. I switched on the first side of *Murder Must Advertise*, the fact that I had read it before and had heard most of it on the radio at home, only added to my pleasure and made it possible to ration myself to two out of the four sides. At 10.30pm I changed the tape to *Poetry Please* and fell asleep to the voice of Jim Piggott-Smith reciting *The Deserted Village*.

The British High Commission holds a Christmas party every year for the VSOs to which the other British residents in Freetown are invited. I was thrilled to open my formal invitation, delivered, of course, by hand to the main clinic. It was a truly memorable occasion. The rains were well past and the hamartan wind bearing its pall of red dust from the Sahara, was still a few weeks away. The rich blue night of the tropics was lit by a million stars and a brilliant moon. The High Commissioner's Residence was high on the bluff, the paved terrace and its encircling lawns surrounded by the gently waving branches of large trees that clothed the steep slope until it merged in the darkness into the outskirts of the city below. The view from the terrace over the top of the tree canopy to the harbour and the ocean far below was breath taking in daylight.

I arrived early enough to be ushered by a broadly smiling policeman to an easily exited parking slot, for which he was rewarded with a suitable 'dash'. I walked into the Residence, large enough but not ostentatiously so, and walked down the stairs to be greeted by the High Commissioner, no need to be burdened by a wrap in this climate. It was pleasant to be greeted personally by some-one who obviously recognised me and had no need to be briefed, then cross the wide room onto the paved area outside, collecting a drink on the way from one of the immaculately uniformed African servants.

There was already a buzz of anticipatory voices and several friends were drinking their wine or fruit juice on the patio while the fireflies darted like shooting stars about the shrubs and trees around us. As the evening wore on I realised that I knew many of the middle aged and older guests and this gave me a sense of belonging albeit transitorily, to this small enclave of expatriates. No doubt this was what the British High Commission parties were all about.

We oldies were not the raison-d'être for this particular party however. The evening was given over to the young. It was a moving experience to see so many men and women, far more than I had anticipated, who were working up-country in schools, hospitals, agricultural and fishery projects and many other outlets I did not even know existed. Dress was, naturally, informal. VSOs do not pack evening dress in their kit when they leave the UK but they looked clean, cool and attractive and were determined to enjoy this evening of good food, free alcohol, cheerful music and plenty of congenial friends with whom to join in the dancing.

I was sitting with my friends, the Copes, watching an enthusiastic rendering of the Gay Gordons.

"It's so sensible to dance in bare feet," I commented. "Look at that girl over there, she could never be so nimble in a pair of trainers or sandals."

"She looks jolly hot all the same. Where do they get their energy from?" said Hilary wistfully, who was already suffering from a debilitating condition which sapped her strength and made exertion an effort.

At length, when my own feet had almost begun to ache in sympathy, the tune came to an end and one of the girls came over to us. She was certainly 'feeling the heat' but had evidently been thoroughly enjoying herself.

"I don't expect you will remember me but I was on a family planning course in Glasgow and you gave some of the lectures. The one I remember best was all about the different types of condoms the prostitutes used at the Drop-in Centre." She introduced herself and said she was working in a hospital up-country.

"I hope what you learnt on the course has been of some use to you in Sierra-Leone? Knowing which condoms are lubricated with nasty tasting spermicides is pretty irrelevant here! What do you actually do?"

"Well, I do most straight-forward surgery, appendices, hernias, caesarian sections and so on. Sometimes more hairy ops if there is no-one else available."

"Are you enjoying it?"

"Oh, yes. It's great. I wouldn't have missed it for anything. I don't know how I'll cope going back to ordinary medicine in the UK when my two years is up next August."

I had no doubt that she would cope very well. She was that kind of girl.

Leona went back to the United States early in December for her well-earned Christmas leave. In addition to clearing out the Aegean stables left by her predecessor, a mess of corruption, mismanagement and incompetence, she had had to cope with the results of the Liberian civil war. The government forces of the late President Doe were supported by most of the other countries in West Africa, particularly Nigeria. After some months, part of a combined West African Peace Keeping Force was assembled in Sierra-Leone and transhipped to Monrovia to fight the rebels. Prince Johnson's faction was marginalised during these manoeuvres. Although a compromise new Acting President was put in place and Monrovia and its immediate hinterland came under his jurisdiction after a cease-fire was arranged, Charles Taylor remained in de-facto control of most of the rest of the country. This included the long western border with Sierra-Leone which provided a completely undefended frontier for undisciplined young men, armed with modern automatic weapons and machetes to cross the frontier. They had become accustomed to killing and rape and taking whatever they wanted at the point of a gun. Sierra-Leone is poor, but it was a sitting duck waiting to be plucked.

The Liberian civil war impinged daily on the lives of Sierra-Leonians and all of us who lived in the capital. Refugees attending our clinics were entitled to free treatment, the cost of which we could claim back from the Red Cross. Many were staying with friends and relatives which meant both families were overcrowded. Native inhabitants were beginning to resent the Liberians who were often better educated, spoke better English and were competing for the few jobs available to the literate. Liberia had been virtually a colony of the United States, although neither party would have called the relationship by this name, but there had been a huge input of American money and know-how poured into the country for over a hundred years. The Medical School was named after John F Kennedy and judging by the knowledge and attitudes of the two doctors I came to know who worked for Marie-Stopes in the last months of my stay, its standards were of the highest calibre.

The American Embassy in Monrovia was very large and remained virtually unscathed by Government forces or by either of the rebel armies. Naturally, nearly all the civilians were evacuated but a skeleton administration stayed behind protected by, I believe, a force of Marines. Inevitably there was a constant stream of visiting firemen of greater or lesser usefulness who used Freetown as their last staging post before Monrovia. They also needed to be accommodated on their way back to the good old US of A after trips that rarely lasted longer than a week and were usually only for two or three days. Leona appeared to be responsible for all those whose missions were remotely connected with aid or refugees.

She had to arrange for their accommodation in one of the three main hotels, and fix the transport, which had to be through the US military as there were no civilian flights in or out of Liberia. She was also expected to meet them, escort them, and entertain them before ensuring their effortless departure back to the relative luxury and comforts of civilisation. I felt angry on her behalf when she might return from a two day visit up-country driving herself over the terrible roads and would have to be ready to go out to dinner and make small talk with some pedantic know-all who thought he knew all the answers after two days in the US embassy in Monrovia.

Leona had generously offered me the use of her self-catering flat in the Bintumani while she was away, an offer I was delighted to accept. Life in my own apartment in Wilkinson Road had become an endurance test I could only survive by imposing myself on my friends at increasingly frequent intervals and I felt more and more embarrassed when they pressed me to accept their hospitality. The flat at the Bintumani had originally been three separate bedrooms with bathrooms en-suite. One remained a bedroom with a connecting door into the sitting room where the intervening wall had virtually been removed to lead into a kitchen/dining room.

Leona had been given many beautiful things when she had been working for the Catholic Aid society in Thailand, Jordan and Jerusalem and she had been able to bring many of her personal possessions with her from the Middle East. There were two exquisitely made patchwork quilts from Thailand on the beds and there were some lovely pictures, pottery and embroidery which made staying there a very real pleasure, quite apart from all the mod-cons. Although there was a modern stainless steel sink unit, the only means of cooking was her own microwave oven. I had never used one of these before and I found it ironic that I should learn to do so in Sierra-Leone! In typical American fashion, Leona had all the necessary equipment, a drawer full of tea-towels and two recipe books (including instructions) for the oven.

The sitting-room had a balcony which was wide enough to accommodate an upright chair without discomfort and long enough to hold three seats in a row. It was here that we used to sit with our Star beers on the top of the parapet in front of us and enjoy the incomparable view for half an hour as the sun set and it grew suddenly dusk, before we went down to drive to whichever nearby restaurant we fancied. Her flat was four floors above the scrub covered ground which sloped down to the inlet. The beach curved sharply round connecting the tiny peninsula opposite by a narrow neck barely wider than the road which led to the Cape Sierra Hotel and the palm and brush covered hummock with a small working lighthouse at its Northern extremity. From where we sat we could see far beyond the Cape Sierra and the lighthouse to the limitless Atlantic and the ships lying in the roads waiting for the tide, or the Port Authority, to allow them into, or away from, Freetown harbour. During the rainy season the sunsets were sometimes spectacular – red, gold, violet, towering masses of thunderous black edged with silver against glimpses of duck egg blue with nothing but the sea meeting the horizon in an almost imperceptible line.

The rains were nearly over now and the sunsets less spectacular but still worth watching and I was going to be able to enjoy them every day for five weeks. The power came on pretty regularly at 6.00 and I could cook a hot meal in the microwave with the balcony door open to allow the fresh breeze from the sea to cool the room. I could read or write letters or listen to a tape or the radio without using up my precious batteries and I could go to bed in an air-conditioned room knowing I would be able to sleep soundly until, inevitably, my bladder woke me up when I had the choice of three bathrooms from which to choose. I was certainly going to lead the life of Riley.

On the Thursday before Christmas I did my usual session at the Collegiate School Road clinic. There were fewer patients than usual, probably because people were spending any money they had on the festivities, whether Christian, Muslim or of other beliefs. There is a remarkable tolerance and lack of bigotry in Sierra-Leone which could teach Glaswegians a lot, and public holidays based on religious feast days like Christmas are enjoyed by all. 'Midnight Picnics' over the festive season are enjoyed by everyone and children of every faith expect some extra treat because it is Christmas. As I had finished before 1 o'clock I decided I would drive into town and post some letters in the central post office, the only reliable letterbox in the capital. I always used air letters with no enclosures and they usually arrived, often surprisingly quickly. I was also going to treat myself to a toasted cheese sandwich and an ice-cold 7-Up at the British council.

I was sitting down sinking my teeth into the delicious crispness of the toast when an English voice asked, "Please could you tell me where I can buy a stamp and post a letter?" A short middle-aged perspiring and rather bedraggled looking woman was standing looking down at me with a trace of desperation in her eyes.

"Of course, but do sit down and cool off a bit. Would you like a Sprite or a Coke or something?" This she refused having already had a drink but she collapsed gratefully into the other chair when I told her that I was going to the post office myself and would gladly give her a lift. Naturally I was intrigued to find out what she was doing in Freetown and was astonished when she said she was on holiday.

"But nobody has a holiday in Freetown unless they are staying with close relatives or friends!" I exclaimed.

"That's what I've found out now I've got here. I've always enjoyed rather off-beat holidays and I'm single with no ties so I can please myself. I'm a social worker in London. Sixteen years ago I was working in a residential home for children and a Sierra-Leonian woman worked there with me. We kept vaguely in touch through mutual friends but I haven't actually seen her for more than twelve years," she went on to explain.

"Then early in November I got a letter from her asking me to come for Christmas. I had no plans to go anywhere else and had some leave due to me, so, I thought, why not? Booked my ticket and came out, not without a bit of strife over my visa though." The almost blatant request for extra funds to facilitate the swift processing of the paper work by the office in London had made her very indignant but she had managed to obtain the necessary document in time for her departure without further payment. This experience had left a slightly nasty taste in her mouth which even so, had not prepared her for the horrors of Lungi airport. I had found it daunting enough accompanied by a native Sierra-Leonian and being met by our own driver and transport. There was nobody to meet Corinne and she had to battle her way through the jungle of passport, currency, health and customs, collect her one small suitcase and find the KLM bus while fending off all the over-eager arms trying to take it out of her hand and into a waiting taxi for extortionate transport to Freetown.

To Corinne it had been the beginning of a nightmare in which she was still living. Her hostess had sent someone to meet her at the bus terminal in the city. It was nearly midnight and she had been travelling for eighteen hours. She was driven to an address in the suburb of Murray Town, and the last part of the road was very rough, as I came to learn. She arrived eventually at the house, a modest single storey dwelling opening virtually onto the street and close to its neighbours on either side. It was immediately apparent that Mrs Darling, her hostess, was more interested in what Corinne had brought with her than in the details of the uncomfortable journey. She had sent a letter explaining that she was planning to have a big party for her seventieth birthday and asking

Corinne to bring a 20lb turkey, sausages and all the other trimmings of the traditional English Christmas and had indicated that a fairly substantial personal gift would be expected as well. Corinne had responded by bringing the bird, but 12lbs was all she felt able to manage in addition to the sausages and so on. The immediate welfare of these perishable meats was the priority, which was not perhaps unreasonable in a temperature of 85°F plus and 90% humidity but she had not expected to be harangued about her failure to bring a heavier turkey. As soon as the goodies were stored in the deep freeze, she was shown into a small room containing a narrow bed and an upright chair, the door was shut and that was it. No refreshment, not even a drink was offered but she hoped for better things in the morning. Unhappily she still had to survive the night. Although exhausted, sleep was virtually impossible as the building next door, literally six feet from her head, housed a disco from which loud pounding rhythms poured out into the darkness until five am.

Morning did not bring better things. She was an alien in an alien world and did not understand that many of the things she took exception to were not directed against her personally but were normal practice in a middle class Sierra-Leonian household. Mrs Darling had a car in the garage next to her house but it was never used, probably because it had no fuel. All food and household goods were kept locked up and only Mrs Darling had the keys. This was to prevent petty thieving by any of the numerous individuals who wandered in and out of the house at all times of the day and evening. Corinne felt infuriated when she found she had to ask for toilet paper and was issued with two sheets after the appropriate cupboard had been ostentatiously unlocked so that all the casual visitors knew what she had asked for. She was never introduced to these people who, naturally talked amongst themselves in Krio which Corinne could not follow.

About two in the morning of the second night the disco was blaring out as before and she had such a splitting headache that she decided to take two paracetamol and make herself a cup of tea. She crept out of her room using a small pocket torch she had brought with her, and opened the kitchen door. Immediately there was a tremendous squawking and flapping which intensified as soon as she moved further into the room.

"And what do you think you're doing in my kitchen after midnight?" Mrs Darling was shaking with rage. "You've no business to be in here disturbing my hens and my ducks who should be left to sleep in peace. Go back to your bed at once." Upon which she firmly locked the kitchen door and continued to do so every night for as long as Corinne stayed there.

On the third day Corinne was desperate and felt she must get out of the house and see something of Freetown. She had neither guide nor map but she was able to ask her way to the town centre without difficulty as most city-dwellers understand a little English. She had arrived at the British Council after walking nearly three miles in the heat and humidity of mid-day. No wonder she looked hot and a little dishevelled.

We went to the post office together and then I drove her back to the house in Murray Town. I was introduced to a less than enthusiastic Mrs Darling who did not invite me in. I had arranged to pick Corinne up the following evening to take her out to an ocean-side restaurant and show her that there was a lot more to Freetown than dirt roads and discos.

We went to Harry's and had a delicious seafood meal under the rustling palms while the tide gently lapped its way nearly to our feet as we sat beside the lagoon. Poor Corinne, it was then time for me to drive her back to Murray Town, not a journey I was looking forward to over the ridges and, hopefully, round, the worst of the pot-holes in the dark, with the ever present knowledge that a puncture was all too likely. The big party was the next day and she felt she must be present as that had been the main excuse for getting her out to Sierra-Leone. The day after that was Christmas day.

Later I dropped her off and waited until I heard the bolts withdrawn and a muttered grumble as she was let into the house. It was only 9.30pm so there was no need for either of us to feel guilty.

Christmas Day dawned. My family had sent two tapes via the Marie-Stopes DHL bag as well as a Colin Baxter diary for 1991. I had refrained from listening to the family greetings with considerable difficulty and decided to wait until I was up, dressed and fed before indulging myself. I put the other tape into Leona's cassette player, the hotel generator was still going in honour of the holiday, and I made a cup of tea and ate my toast and marmalade to the angelic strains of Christmas carols sung by cathedral choirs from all over England. When I had washed up and put everything away (I conformed to Leona's convential standards of tidiness when I stayed in her flat) I relaxed in an easy chair and settled down to enjoy the rather chaotic messages and chatter from my children and grand-children. At 10 o'clock I left, but remembered to leave a message at reception to allow entry into the flat by any English lady that enquired for me.

I had been invited to join a small party from the British High

Commission, two of whom rented a beach house near Tokay. I drove up to the BHC compound and soon three four-wheel drive vehicles loaded, not only with people but with all the food and paraphernalia for a traditional English Christmas dinner, set off for the 'picnic'. The site of the beach house was so like a picture on the front of a travel brochure that it was difficult to believe it was real.

The table was set with a festive cloth and candles; cutlery and wine glasses completed the setting for the feast.

I must admit that while all the preparations were going on I was enjoying an idyllic bathe. A path led from the knoll down to a rocky pool washed smooth by the constant action of the tides. It was deep enough to float with one's posterior anchored on a rounded boss on the bottom while the waves poured in over the natural weir fronting the ocean and then retreated, lifting one gently up and down on the swell. Two other guests were enjoying the pleasures of the pool, a husband and wife who had been living in Liberia on a huge Chinese-owned rubber plantation. Richard had been the manager and Margaret had been responsible for organising the school and hospital for the local employees. They had had to flee at very short notice and leave all but their most personal small possessions behind when the civil war brought Charles Taylor's marauding trigger happy 'troops' into their district. The three of us basked in the warm buoyant water, talking of books and food and many things besides life's immediate problems.

We went back to the beach hut and I changed into a loose top and skirt having no desire to expose my too, too solid flesh to the common gaze while we were enjoying our Christmas dinner. The candles were lit, the crackers pulled, the paper hats donned and we all enjoyed turkey and the trimmings (even the sprouts were in the best British boarding house tradition, small, hard, grey and smelly), Christmas pudding and white sauce, and, in common with many Christmases we had all enjoyed before, nobody had any room for the mince-pies. We drank to 'absent friends' and to the future in deliciously chilled white wine from the cold box or pleasantly 'breathing' red poured from the open bottles while, in the background, my tape of cathedral choristers reminded us nostalgically of holidays in England, long ago.

I got back to the Bintumani about 6.00 and found my key was no longer at reception. I went up to the flat and knocked on the door and was not surprised to find Corinne was there before me. She had found it impossible to stay on with Mrs Darling, who, by this time, would no longer speak to her. She had walked from Murray town with her toothbrush in her handbag but had been able to relax and recuperate in the relative cool and quiet of the hotel.

She slept the night on the settee, both of us preferring not to have to share a room when there was a choice. The next day was Boxing Day and I had written to my family telling them that I would stay in all morning and sending them the telephone number of the hotel. I was really looking forward to being able to speak, at least to some of them, for the first time in four months.

Corinne and I had just finished a leisurely breakfast when there was a knock at the door. It was an Irishman from the Mami-Yoko whom I had successfully treated for scabies on his backside which he had picked up in his flight from Liberia. However, it was not a recurrence of his itch but a message from Margaret to say that Richard was ill and could I possibly go and see him? It appeared that he was vomiting repeatedly and, of course, I would have to visit him. He was lying back on the pillows looking very grey and drawn. His eyes were shut but opened when I sat on the edge of the bed and spoke to him.

"Have you got a pain any where?"

"No, my head aches a bit but I've no pain in my stomach."

"Had any diarrhoea?"

"No, just this frightful nausea."

I noticed he kept his head unnaturally still, and indeed hardly moved his eyes from my face. I put my hand behind his head and gently lifted it forwards so that his chin was touching his chest. He protested, but not because it hurt the back of his neck as it would have done if he had meningitis but because it brought on a wave of nausea and retching. I examined his abdomen but it was soft and unresisting with no tenderness to indicate any inflammatory process going on inside.

"I'm so giddy when I try to stand and go to the lavatory. Everything just goes round and I lose my balance," he explained.

I asked him to focus on the end of my index finger which I held about six inches in front of his nose.

"Now follow it with your eyes, keeping your head still." I moved it slowly to the left for about a foot and held it there watching his eyes carefully. They both moved sideways with the finger tip but once at the extremity of the lateral field they flicked back halfway, returned more slowly to the left and flicked uncontrollably back to the middle again. This repetitive eye movement is called nystagmus and indicates a severe upset in the mechanism of balance.

"I'm pretty sure you've got something called acute labyrinthitis, it's nasty but not serious and usually clears up on its own in a few days." I explained that I did not know the cause but as it sometimes occurred in small epidemics it was probably due to a 'virus', but I was sure there were no antibiotics which would do any good. However, sometimes pills used to treat motion sickness did help the nausea and these might be available in the small pharmacy in the hotel.

"The most important thing is to keep still and not try to get out of bed unless you've absolutely got to. Don't worry about eating, but try and get some fluids down in small sips at a time."

Margaret walked with me along the corridor from their room. I knew she was still very worried even though her immediate fears of some serious heart or abdominal condition had receded, because they were booked on a flight to London in six days time. This was their first 'home' leave for two years and the first break they would be enjoying since escaping from Liberia. They had appointments in London to report to the company chiefs to give a personal account of the situation as far as was possible and then they had booked a holiday in Madeira after staying with friends and family for a few days in England. All these plans were now in jeopardy but I reassured her that there was every chance that Richard would be well enough to travel and there was no point in making any changes of plan at this early stage.

"I'll be back around tea-time," I said as I left her in the foyer, remembering the last case of labyrinthitis I had seen which had taken nearly a month to clear up.

When I got back to the Bintumani the girl at reception told me that a phone call had come for me from the UK but she had not been able to put it through to my room as there was a fault in the internal lines. I asked her to send one of the porters to fetch me without delay if it happened again but, as I found out later, nobody else even managed to get a connection to Freetown and I was doomed to disappointment. I had arranged with the family to try in the morning only so after lunch I was free to take Corinne back to Mrs Darling's to collect her things. Neither of us was looking forward to the expedition and I had visions of either not being able to get into her house at all or of the suitcase being thrown out onto the street accompanied by a stream of vituperative abuse. In the event the transaction was carried out with icy politeness and everyone's dignity remained intact.

I drove Corinne to my apartment in Wilkinson Road. I did not bother to drive into the compound as her suitcase was not heavy now it had been relieved of the extras brought over for her ex-hostess. I had informed my landlord's wife that a friend would be staying in the flat for the next week or so. I was glad it was Mrs Brown and not her husband who answered the door, he could be a surly and difficult man to deal with at times. We walked down the concrete slope at the side of the house picking our way among the rivulets of water that leaked from the waste-pipe and spread over the cement in a fan as it reached the flat terrace in front of my door. As we rounded the corner of the house the two watchmen and the house-boy quickly turned their naked backs.

They were washing themselves at the stand-pipe in the yard as they always did, and as I was away, were naturally not expecting two white women to interrupt their ablutions. I thought no more about it until Corinne remarked that it was a good job she was not a shrinking violet and, although she was over fifty and unmarried, this did not mean she was unfamiliar with living versions of Michael Angelo's *David*. I unlocked the three padlocks and showed her all that was necessary. Of course there was no power but at least there was relative peace and quiet and unlimited toilet paper! We had brought some food supplies from the Bintumani and I had pointed out a little local store within easy walking distance where she could go tomorrow when the holiday would be over.

It was back to work the next day but the clinics at Ports and Kissy were light and I had time to go to Choitrams, the city centre supermarket and choose some supplies for a small party I planned to hold in the flat on the Sunday between Christmas and New Year.

I called in again to see Richard, I knew he was improving because he was already proving a demanding patient and Margaret was finding it increasingly difficult to find ways of keeping him amused. He still found reading for any length of time upset his balance but he could get to the lavatory with her help without falling or actually vomiting. The next day was Saturday and I made some more purchases for my party the next day, in particular buying oranges, pineapple, pawpaw and bananas for a fresh fruit salad and the cherry-sized local tomatoes, 'Irish' potatoes and onions for a savoury one. I had managed to find some long thin continental type sausages in Choitrams, which, cut into short lengths and heated in the microwave and impaled on a stick (a box of which I found among Leona's kitchen equipment) made excellent cocktail bites.

After lunch I went to see Richard hoping to find him much better but he had, in fact, relapsed. It was his own fault, he had felt almost recovered and so had insisted on using his lap-top computer on his knees in bed to try and complete some business before he went back to England. The concentration and repeated but restricted eye movements had brought about a return of the nausea and he was lying back feeling lousy and very sorry for himself while Margaret was having great difficulty in restraining herself from saying 'I told you so'.

The party the next day went very well. I had invited all my friends who were free to come and arranged for the Shepherds to pick up Corinne from the flat – about a dozen in all, which was as many as the flat could comfortably accommodate. As it was, some people were sitting on cushions on the floor. I was delighted to be able to show even such minimal hospitality to those who had been so good to me. Most of my European guests had not met Sylvia before but, even so, she seemed to find a mutual acquaintance with everyone she spoke to, which not only demonstrated her social skills but underlined how small the professional and business class is in Freetown, regardless of the varied ethnic backgrounds.

This celebration marked the end of the festive season for me and it was back to work on the Monday for all of us.

Richard did recover sufficiently to be able to travel back to the UK on his scheduled flight although I had to write a letter stating that, in my opinion, flying would not cause a serious deterioration in his condition. I confess my knowledge of the effects of altitude (in a pressurised aircraft) on acute labyrinthitis was nil but on common-sense grounds I could not see that it should make any difference and I felt it was important from every point of view that they should return to the UK as soon as possible, where, if Richard was going to continue to be unwell, at least the full range of medical care was available and their family would be there to give support.

Chapter 6 - January
O Yan Look Wae You Small En Fat . . .

EARLY IN JANUARY, I RECEIVED A NOTICE
from the Post Office that informed me that there was a parcel waiting
for me to collect. I was quite excited. Had someone managed to send me
a Christmas present which had miraculously survived the tampering
hands of the postal staff?

The following Monday I finished my duties at Adelaide Street and
went into the city centre. The parcel repository was down on the water
front and I made my way accordingly. I parked the car in the pock-marked
street and approached the building on foot. It was a very large Victorian
structure which must have been handsome in its heyday and, even now,
it was still impressive. There was a wide flight of steps leading up to a
pair of imposing double doors which were shut. On either side of this
central stair there were matching but narrower flights which led to two
single doors. All three flights spanned an open drain, six feet across and
eight feet deep, which smelt and looked as though it collected all the
sewage in Freetown. Less than a hundred yards beyond it discharged
into the sea. The stench was nauseating and I hurried up the main flight
to find the doors firmly locked. I retreated over the sewer, and scanned
the front of the building.

A small dirty piece of paper was attached to the left-hand pillar of
the double doors. I mounted the steps again. "Closed 12.30 – 1.30". It
was now 12.50. It was too hot to sit in the car but the smell made it
impossible to wait where I was. I found a shady seat on a wall, far enough
away to allow me to breathe through my nose without distaste, and at
1.30, strolled back. All the doors were open – no doubt the inhabitants
of the building were inured to the stench and appreciated a sea breeze. I
went up the central steps into a huge cavernous warehouse with a long
mahogany counter, at least three feet wide, preventing further advance.
It stretched into the semi-darkness on either side. A wizened but very
self-important official was standing behind it.

"You must not come in this door, you must come in that one," and he gesticulated firmly to his right. I apologised and went out into the unrelenting heat, taking a deep breath of the less polluted air inside before I had to cross the stinking moat. I advanced once more, this time up the left hand steps. The same gentleman stood behind what I could now see, was the same counter.

"What do you want?"

"I have had this paper to tell me there is a parcel here for me," I held out the official form. He scrutinised it carefully.

"Proof of identity," he said. Luckily I had my driving licence in my wallet.

"OK, you must come with me." I looked at the solid mahogany. "You must go outside and come in the main doors."

I knew better than to protest, and dutifully went outside and once more climbed up the stairs and went through the double doors. There he was again, but he had changed his baseball cap for more official headgear, like that of a Salvation Army officer suitably badged and braided. He lifted a flap in the counter and admitted me to the gloomy space behind. It was only then that I appreciated the enormous size of the repository. The roof was the height of a three story building and the internal space was subdivided by huge ranks of shelves reaching into the darkness. It was filthy with the dirt of several decades. As he led me into a relatively open area on the left-hand side, we passed tables piled with packets and parcels that were covered in dust and bird droppings. We stopped at another small table and he sat down behind it and adjusted his uniform cap more firmly on his head.

"Sign here." He had flipped over several dirty sheets on a pad before he found a clean one and then laboriously filled out my details with a short blunt pencil. I signed, using my own biro as he said my signature must be in ink. I would have given it to him but I only had one spare back at the flat, and pens of any kind were difficult to come by. When this ceremony was completed we walked back to the entrance and I was ushered through the raised counter flap.

"Please may I have the parcel now?" I asked meekly.

"Yes, but you must go to the right department. You go in through that door." This time he waved to his left. I was beginning to enjoy this long drawn-out farce and smiled as I said, "Certainly," much to his disgruntled surprise. Down I went and up the other side, which at least made a change. Once inside the right-hand door, there was my friend, back in his baseball cap behind the same long counter which stretched across most of the front of the warehouse. This time he had a small parcel, more of a large packet really, which was the object of all these manoeuvres. It said 'medical supplies' on the outside and had been posted in October by a colleague in Glasgow. It had been torn open at one end so that the contents could be seen. I delayed opening it properly until I was back in the car. It contained pregnancy testing kits. Two of the original ten were missing – no doubt the thieves could not understand their purpose and saw no resale value in them. Technically they were now past their sell-by date but the remaining eight were still functional, and we made good use of them in the clinics over the next few weeks.

As far as I could see or hear my two-capped friend was the sole inhabitant of the Parcel Repository. Its size made one aware that there had been a time when such a large and imposing structure had been necessary to accommodate the volume of postal traffic that came in and out of Freetown. Ships had called regularly carrying the Royal Mail and post from all the other corners of the earth. The hundreds of yards of shelving would have been in daily use and probably hundreds of people were employed. It is not like that now.

I moved back to the flat at the beginning of the second week in January. Corinne Shamrock had returned thankfully to London and Leona Donahue, perhaps less thankfully, to Freetown. A ship had arrived with Calor gas cylinders amongst its cargo so I was now able to cook and my diet became more interesting, although, in the absence of electricity, I found it practical to prepare my evening meal before 6.30pm when it became difficult to see how much soup there was in the pan before the spaghetti was added. While I had been away, my landlord had erected a large concrete hut in the garden which now housed a big generator. In the front of the compound was a tall structure, not unlike a small lighthouse, on which was proudly mounted an enormous television receiving dish. It was placed so that anyone driving past could not fail to notice it and enabled him to tune in to a TV network which was relayed from a station in Bophuthatswana. I was told by Ken that this new piece of apparatus used less than half the power of an air-conditioner. When I told Sylvia of this latest development she decided to make another approach to Mr Brown about the lack of power in my flat. There was no question of asking for a free supply. We were expecting to pay. It only required a cable from the new generator to the flat, a distance of, at most ten yards. He rudely refused.

"You should not have employed a doctor from England," he said.

117

"You should have somebody who could 'beyah' (bear) it. Somebody who is used to the climate and does not need an air-conditioner and who can cook on a coal (charcoal) stove."

"You are the one to talk," she replied, hotly. "What about your own family? They do not 'beyah' it, even though they were born here! There are at least two air-conditioners on in your house every night. I have heard them, and you say you cannot spare Doctor Wilson even enough power to give her light for three hours at night." He was adamant and I never had a power supply from him.

It was good to get back to the more or less weekly evenings out with Leona, and I still enjoyed going to the golf club on Thursdays, not only for the fish and chips, which were very good, but also for the opportunity to meet friends and acquaintances. I soon became aware that there was some extra-golfing activity in the wind. A small group of men would sit outside the club-house with a round of drinks on the table in front of them, earnestly discussing something which, to an uninvolved observer, was obviously becoming increasingly boring to the majority, who would begin to fidget, tip their chairs, yawn and even doze off at times.

"What on earth's going on out there?" I asked Hilary Cope.

"Oh, it's the Burns Night Supper committee. Haven't you noticed they're nearly all Scots?"

Sure enough nearly every-one of the eight (or at most ten) Caledonians in Freetown were assembled, with patently varying degrees of enthusiasm and, as is usual in such circumstances, nearly all the work was being done by one individual and his side-kick. Blessed be Saint Andrew, Saint Patrick and Saint George and long may it be before the doubts about the latter's existence percolate through to the College of Heralds. The celebration of their name-days provides expatriate British communities all over the world with sound patriotic excuses to have a party on an official scale. The Scots, as usual, manage to capitalise on their national assets more effectively than the English, (how many English people even know the name of their patron saint, let alone the date on which his festival is celebrated?).

The Scots have two patron saints, the uncanonised one being by far the better known, and wherever two or three are gathered together in January, it is in the name of Robert Burns. There are certain essential ingredients for any Burns' night supper – the whisky, the pipes, the kilts, the haggis – accompanied, of course, by tatties and bashed neeps, those unattractive reminders of the poverty of the Scottish diet in the nineteenth century. But the mind must also be fed along traditional lines. The recitation of *Tam O'Shanter*, the singing of *My Love is Like a Red, Red Rose*, the final *Auld Lang Syne*, are all peripheral to the toast of 'The Immortal Memory' which is supposed to be the tour de force of the evening. 'The Lassies' must be proposed and, as is the custom at all formal dinners, 'The Guests' also.

The committee were having difficulty in finding speakers, not necessarily good or appropriate speakers, but any speakers at all. A distinguished Indian lady doctor eventually agreed, but when she realised that she was expected to give a potted history of Scotland's greatest poet including references to his significance in Sierra-Leone and, if possible, a bawdy quotation or two to encourage the conviviality of the evening, she opted for a combination of 'The Lassies' and 'The Guests'.

I had rashly told Donald MacLeod weeks before that I had once been asked to propose 'The Immortal Memory' at a hospital dinner in Glasgow. The main point of the story had been the problems I had had trying to find a reference book from which to cull the basic facts. As usual, I had left it to the last minute, or at least the weekend before. I had popped in to the local public library, not anticipating any difficulty, only to find there were no books on Burns on the shelves. I had asked the librarian where all the Burns' books were.

"There's always a rush on them at this time of year, all the schools do Burns projects and all the books about him just melt off the shelves. They'll be back by the end of next week," she had added cheerfully. Of course, I should have realised that I was not the only one seeking to refresh my all too mortal memory.

There had been nothing for it but to dip my hand in my pocket and go to a book shop. My first choice was *Burns Night, All You Need To Know*. Amongst chapters on how to calculate the amount of whisky that would be required and how to deal with the haggis was one on 'How to Choose the Speaker'.

Unfortunately Donald remembered this story and two weeks before the coming event, he somewhat sheepishly asked me if I would fill the breech. I agreed, on condition that we could find some work of reference to provide the necessary skeleton framework for the toast. Needless to say, I had not included the *Complete Works of Robert Burns* (including a biography) in the luggage I had brought out to West Africa. I had been tens of kilos overweight, with nearly a suitcase full of books and audio-tapes, pregnancy testing kits, my sphygmomanometer for taking blood pressures, a hammer, nails, sellotape, paper, a mosquito net and everything that the Mother in Swiss Family Robinson might have carried in her carpet bag, which might come in useful.

The next day was Sunday and Ken Shepherd drove me in his Land-Rover up, down and across the maze of unmade roads cutting into the hillside between the British High Commission Compound and Wilkinson Road searching for Douglas, the Chief of the Caledonian Society, under whose aegis the Burns Night Supper was being organised. Eventually we did find his house, but he was not there, and we had to leave a note with his steward, suitably accompanied by a 'dash' to try and ensure its safe delivery. Two days later I received a message via the Shepherds, to meet Douglas at the club-house that evening. Sure enough, there he was, and he greeted me warmly.

"I've got just the thing for you," he said, and produced *Burns Night, All You Need To Know* in triumph from his brief-case. He must have seen my face fall, for he added quickly, "Of course, I've got the *Complete Works* as well, but I thought that might be a little heavy for you."

I assured him that the larger volume was all that I needed, and refreshed with a Star beer, I drove back to the flat to start my homework.

The MacLeods had asked me to stay with them over the festive weekend. This made it much easier for me to do the last minute revision of my script, which I always require, as I could read my notes by electric light rather than candle-power. Jane's major contribution to the occasion was twenty-two bottles of atholl brose, a delicious concoction of whisky, honey and oatmeal which she brewed herself. Each table was to be given one free with the compliments of the Caledonian Society. As Jane much preferred the company of a few personal friends to a big formal occasion, and as she was a vegetarian and rarely touched alcohol, I realised that under her gentle and unemphatic manner there must be a strong sense of national identity which led her into spending so much time and effort supporting an occasion she would have much preferred to have missed.

About half an hour before we were due to leave all the lights went out and the air-conditioners stopped. There had obviously been a major fault in the generator which supplied the compound. Jane and Donald were not the only company employees to occupy a house inside its walls. The steward of the other family had managed to blow a main fuse, which had to be replaced by torch-light. When the spare fuse was sought, it was no longer there, and the only replacement was at the company factory in the East end of the town. Donald set off without delay to collect the vital part, probably a round trip of no more than ten miles but it meant driving through the middle of the city on bad roads and with unaccountable traffic. A long delay seemed inevitable. Jane had just washed her hair when the power failed and was still in her kimono. I had showered and changed into a caftan, the nearest I could get in Sierra-Leone to an evening dress, but I had been hoping for a last minute glance at my notes. More important than all our personal inconveniences was the fact that the atholl brose was still standing, carefully packed in the Mitsubishi, waiting to be carried to the Bintumani Hotel.

Miraculously, Donald was back in little over half an hour and it was not long before we were able to set off. The quickest way was down the steep hill to Congo Cross, then along Wilkinson Road to the fork for Aberdeen and the Bintumani. We were, or rather would have been, in sight of the turn off, when the vehicles in front slowed and then came to a halt. It was not difficult to see what was causing the obstruction, an enormous articulated truck was trying to back into the yard of a small but pricey supermarket which catered for Western and Lebanese tastes. It had become impacted across the main road, with its front end well inside the open gates of the compound opposite. There was a great deal of shouting and gesticulation and there was not a chance that it could be extracted in the foreseeable future. We did a U-turn and retraced our wheels, back to Congo Cross up the 1 in 6 hill, left at the top, along the crest until we joined the descending loops of Spur Road and bypassed the obstruction by going the long way round via the beach.

Late as we were, we were not too late to arrange for the distribution of the atholl brose to each of the long tables set out under the palm trees. A pleasant breeze ruffled the surface of the swimming pool which, not infrequently, was the only source of water for non-drinking purposes available to the hotel guests and residents. When local fishermen got tired of going out to sea, they preferred the easier option of dynamiting the fish in the shallow waters where the lagoon merged into the ocean. Unfortunately, this was where the mains water pipe was laid, connecting the Aberdeen peninsula to the mainland. The pipe was frequently damaged, to the frustration of the managements of the three big hotels and the considerable inconvenience of their inhabitants. Tonight the water supply was intact, and the Bintumani had ensured that there was enough fuel for their huge generator for this festive occasion. Fairy lights hung in garlands from the trees and the tables were decorated with tropical flowers and coloured napkins.

We were greeted by Douglas in his presidential role, suitably attired for a similar outdoor occasion in his native Scotland, kilt (eight yards of wool plaid deeply pleated), sporran, black dress jacket (with silver buttons), waistcoat, white dress shirt and black patent leather shoes. The other six native Scotsmen were similarly dressed, although two or three wore hairy Harris tweed instead of broad-cloth. One brave and sensible man wore his kilt with a white shirt only and the sleeves rolled up. "Bully for you," I thought to myself.

The worst sufferer was the young piper, flown out specially by British Airways (there was rarely a full complement of paying passengers and a few months later British Airways withdrew from the Freetown route). He had not only to wear the full panoply of Highland dress, but also had to cope with the plaid, a broad three yard long piece of tartan cloth designed to enable him to emulate Prince Charles Edward Stewart and sleep out in the heather in mid winter on Rannoch Moor, without freezing to death. He was not as unhappy as one might have thought, although he was certainly sweating and was extremely hot. He thought the whole thing was a great lark, especially as he had not a drop of Scottish blood in his veins and lived in north London where he played in a police band. No doubt his enjoyment was enhanced by the presence of his girl friend who had been invited to accompany him.

I remember little of the meal except that Jane found nearly all of it inedible, not only the overcooked chicken drumsticks which revolted her vegetarian palate. The haggis was piped in and the young Londoner had his moment of glory, but all too soon it was time to toast 'The Immortal Memory'.

"Chieftan, Your Excellencies, Scots, Sierra-Leonians, Sassenachs, Mongrels like myself, Ladies and Gentlemen, Robert Burns was born in an insignificant corner of Scotland in 1759 and died thirty seven years later. . . " I spoke of his humble origin and his rise to fame, quoting from some of his better known verse and some that is not so well known."

> There's Sophie tight
> A lassie bright
> Beside a handsome fortune,
> Wha canna win her in a night
> Has little art in courtin.

I was anxious to include some local colour and with the help of the English department at St Joseph's Secondary School, I attempted to render *To a mouse, on turning up in her nest with the plough, November 1785*. The Scots version reads,

> Wee sleekit cowran timrous beastie
> Oh, what a panics in thy breastie wi bickering brattle
> I wad be loathe to rin and chase thee wi murdring pattle.

As I said, "Perhaps, if Burns had been a Sierra-Leonian we would
have had this version in Krio,
> O Yah Look wae you small en fat
> You dae make plenty noise because you dae fraid me
> De fraid make you confuse
> You nor for run a way
> Ar nor go lek for run ata you
> Wit dis tik for kill you.

I thought this translation was beautifully done and caught the essence
of the verse with great sensitivity. The audience might have been able to
appreciate both versions better if I had more skill in speaking any
language other than my mother tongue, but at least both versions were
so anglicised that most of my listeners probably understood more than
if I had been fluent in either old Scots or Krio.

It was good when it was over and I could enjoy a last quaff of atholl
brose, knowing that I was going back to the hospitality of the MacLeods
for the rest of the weekend and had no worries about having to drive
myself home. The evening ended with some vigorous Scottish country
dancing which meant palms were very sweaty when it came to *Auld Lang
Syne*, but there is nothing like a bit of shared perspiration to induce a
fellow feeling.

Ever since I started visiting the Blind School regularly I had been
concerned about the general health of the students. Probably they all
had worms, and most would be anaemic in consequence, with little in
their diet to compensate for the daily micro-loss of blood. Hookworms,
threadworms, roundworms and tapeworms were all part of the parasitic
fauna to be found in the intestines of untreated children. One of the
older boys had come to the Collegiate School Road clinic asking for
treatment for "urrm in the belly" because he had vomited the night before
and a large roundworm had had to be pulled out of his throat.

At first I had thought of obtaining stool specimens, and even blood
samples from every student to establish a firm diagnosis, but the logistics
of this were formidable. In practise it was not possible for each child to
produce a stool sample into a previously labelled container with a narrow
neck, with minimal adult supervision, and without being able to see. To
obtain blood samples from forty children would have entailed mass
transport to the hospital laboratory or my taking a test from each one,
single-handed, both of which were impossible. The obvious solution was
to treat all the students for worms, and follow this up with a course of

iron for a month. At that time the only anti-helminthic (anti-worm) treatment we had, involved a single dose of tablets taken first thing in the morning, the number varying between three and six according to the weight of the recipient.

I knew that compliance would be the main problem. The school had now appointed a pleasant motherly woman to be the house-mother and I explained my plans to both Mrs Barrie and the Headmaster, who were enthusiastic, especially when I emphasised that the treatment would be free and that children of staff would be included in the regime.

I could not put the plan into effect immediately as we had to have sufficient stocks of the right medicaments in store without endangering our clinic supplies. Fortunately a new order was due in, and the drugs arrived within two weeks. Mrs Barrie told me that the students had their breakfast at 7.30 in the morning and I was there, waiting for them, the next day. I stood in the dusty dining room in the half light of dawn with the bare, not very clean, trestle tables in three parallel lines across the room. As the children came in, they went to the long serving hatch and were given a plastic mug of water and a chunk of bread. Even Oliver Twist would have felt hard done by. They sat at the tables according to their age, and so it was easy for me to put two or four or six anti-worm tablets into a held-out hand.

"Put them in your mouth and take a drink of water to help you swallow them," I said, and waited and watched to make sure they did. Fortunately none of the children appeared to have any difficulty, even the six year olds taking their two tablets without protest.

The remainder of the treatment depended on Mrs Barrie. Each of the older students was to have three iron tablets a day, the middle school needed two and the juniors, one. I gave her one of the large wide-mouthed containers which held a thousand sugar coated ferrous gluconate tablets. Medically, it would have been preferable to give them another preparation which was better utilised by the body, but the gluconate tablets were very like smarties and were easy to get out of the container with a tablespoon. Dispensing over seventy pills a day for a month required a high degree of commitment on the house-mother's part, and I wanted to make the task as easy as possible. It would have been almost impossible for her to have done it, in the short time the children were assembled at meal times, if the tablets had been less easy to handle. At the end of a fortnight I handed over the second container of a thousand tablets. I would like to say that there was a dramatic improvement in the health of the boys and girls at the school after this mass therapy, but I doubt if an outsider would have noticed any difference. The Headmaster told me that the children were naughtier than they had been, and that was as good an indication of their raised haemoglobins as I would ever know. The Russian doctor was due to go on leave in the near future, much to my relief. We had improved the worst of the hygiene and cross-infection problems by having a half day of in-service training for all the clinical staff, ostensibly concentrating on the risks of AIDS. The couches were now covered by a sheet of plastic under the buttocks and nurses, swabbing away contaminating material, used a suitable antiseptic lotion and wore gloves to do it. The suction syringes, used to perform terminations of pregnancy, were changed after each patient and we now had an autoclave working for an hour at the end of each clinic in Collegiate School Road when the generator was on.

What we had not been able to change was my colleague's attitude to her work and her treatment of her patients. She had been sent on two courses overseas at different times, to learn the techniques of abortion under local anaesthesia and how to perform female sterilisation by the 'mini-lap' method, using no general anaesthetic. She had made full use of the first course, not only when she was employed by Marie-Stopes, but also in her consulting room in the town centre. There was nothing wrong in this, especially as she only worked for us in the mornings, but there was a mounting body of evidence that she was virtually blackmailing patients to see her privately rather than have the operation done at Collegiate. It was easy enough for her to do this as all women wanting a termination had to see her prior to the procedure. No nurse was in the cubicle and our emphasis on privacy and confidentiality precluded the possibility of changing the routine and 'planting' one in with her. Staff who were involved in checking the patients out, began to notice that it was increasingly likely that a proportion of the patients booked in for operation left without having it done.

Then a woman complained. She said the doctor had told her she would get better treatment if she came to see her in her rooms, where the patient would have to pay a much higher fee. The distraught woman said she had no more money, and asked the receptionist what she should do. Another ploy was to take a second fee from the patient when she was doing the preliminary examination in the cubicle prior to operation. The extra money was demanded to ensure that it was done as quickly and painlessly as possible. She still used no local anaesthetic, although supplies were now available, and her manner was less caring than that of most abattoir attendants. She had been actively obstructive as far as the mini-lap programme was concerned and no real progress had been made. A suitable operating table had been donated by my fellow family planning doctors in Scotland. This was a great improvement on the old one, not only for abdominal operations in the future, but for menstrual evacuations now. So far it had never been put to its intended use.

A further cause for concern was that I now had proof that the doctor was not only prescribing inappropriate treatment but using drugs which could do positive harm. A patient attended the small clinic in Aberdeen which was near to her home. She had 'joined family planning' at Collegiate and been started on the pill. Every month she had been troubled by bleeding in the middle of the packet of pills and this had worried her greatly. She went back to the clinic and was referred by the Sister to the Russian doctor who examined her and said she needed an injection followed by a course of pills for three days. This appeared to cure the problem but it recurred the next month, and as she had now discovered that Marie-Stopes had a session once a week in Aberdeen where she lived, she had come to have the treatment again.

Once we asked her the right questions and obtained a proper history the diagnosis was easy, but the treatment was a complete mystery.

I asked Rebecca to translate my questions and the woman's replies into Krio, and visa-versa, as I needed to know exactly what had happened.

"You started the first packet of pills on the fifth day of your period?" She nodded. "Did you ever forget to take any?"

"Oh, no Doctor. I never forgot one."

"That's very good, but when do you take your pills, at night when you go to bed?"

"Sometimes at night but it depends on my husband. . . "

"What do you mean?"

"Well my husband doesn't know I am using family planning and I have to hide the pills. I can only take them at night if he goes to sleep first, otherwise I have to wait until he goes out in the morning."

"So sometimes you take them at night and sometimes not until the middle of the next day?"

"That's right Doctor, but I never forget them."

"I'm sure you don't, but this bleeding you are having is because you are not taking them at the same time every day. You don't HAVE to take them at night, you could take them in the middle of the day if that would suit you better?"

Rebecca listened and translated all this with great interest. When the patient had gone, reassured that she did not need any more expensive medicine and that she could cure the problem herself now she knew what was wrong, Rebecca said, "I didn't know that if you don't take the pills regularly it causes bleeding," she said. "And, I thought you had to take them at night."

"It's a very common problem and gives patients a lot of anxiety, not just in Africa. Unless you explain to them before they start that if there is more than twenty-four hours between each tablet, they may get a little bit of bleeding and if it's as much as half a day, they may have a full 'period', especially in the second half of the packet."

"I've seen lots of women who've had bleeding and most of them stop the pill because they think it isn't agreeing with them."

"Well, now you know it is a very simple problem. It's called 'break-through bleeding' and it's something all you nurses should know about because YOU are the people who can prevent it, and then cure it with the right advice, if it does happen. What worries me is what treatment this lady was given at Collegiate. We must find out and see who prescribed it."

Rebecca made a note of the patient's name and address and we worked out what date, approximately, she must have 'joined family planning' and when she last attended there. Tracing patients without their appointment cards was not easy, as we were only beginning to introduce a system of cross-indexing. Each attender was given the next consecutive number in that year and the flimsy card, even paper, case sheets were filed chronologically. Perhaps it was as well in this instance that there were not nearly as many family planning patients as there were medical, as their notes were filed separately.

Next day, when Rebecca was back at Collegiate she did some detective work at the end of the session, and when I called in during the afternoon, after I had finished at Adelaide Street, she had found the woman's notes. I was horrified to see that she had been given an injection of ergometrine which is sometimes used to stop immediate post-partum bleeding. The tablets, for which she had needed a prescription to be taken to an outside chemist, were for one tablet of ergotamine three times a day, a totally different drug, with a similar sounding name, used in the treatment of migraine. Overdosage can cause serious side effects. I felt I had to inform Sylvia of my disquiet. She was already far from happy about the Russian doctor's attitude and behaviour. The latter resented being under Sylvia's direction, because the Director was a lay person with no medical qualifications, and she was creating problems among the nurses. It would be difficult to sack her.

Sierra-Leone is a small place and every action created a political ripple which was potentially damaging to the relatively new Marie-Stopes organisation. It was a great relief to us all when the doctor failed to return after her annual leave. She had cost Marie-Stopes International many thousands of pounds in terms of payment for training courses and a trip to London to see the central office and enjoy being a tourist for a few days. This had not been enough to buy her loyalty and in this she was not unique. She was the third Sierra-Leonian doctor who had been funded to attend a course out of the country and who had then returned home to practise his, or her, skills exclusively in private practice or to charge the clinic patients a second time, pocketing the covert fee. It was for these reasons that, in Sierra-Leone, Marie-Stopes International's normal practice of employing local doctors in their overseas projects had been broken, and I had been asked to join their project in Freetown.

Towards the end of January Sylvia was approached by another Aid organisation for help in setting up a family planning service within the primary health care project they were hoping to establish up-country. They wanted a detailed estimate of the equipment and supplies needed. I was asked to draw up a list that could then be costed. This was a task which I very much enjoyed, and, as I roughed out the scheme I realised that most of the expense involved in providing a contraceptive service lay in the use of intra-uterine devices.

These demand the provision of an examination couch, special equipment including at least three sets of expensive gynaecological instruments and some facility for sterilising them properly, sterile gloves, a reasonable source of light and a nurse who has been properly trained in the technique of insertion. Medical back-up must be available as clinical complications which can lead to permanent infertility are not unusual. A clinic offering the pill, condoms, foam tablets and the injectable contraceptive, depo-provera could give an excellent service run by properly trained nurses. The only essential equipment needed would be a sphygmomanometer and a stethoscope to monitor the women's blood pressure when using hormonal methods.

The inclusion of inter-uterine contraception multiplied by more than ten the cost of setting up a family planning clinic. This is not justified merely for the sake of the organisation being able to claim that it provides a comprehensive service. In Sierra-Leone, IUDs were the chosen method of less than fiver per cent of contraceptive acceptors attending out Marie-Stopes clinics, in spite of the enthusiasm of the nurses, who enjoyed exercising their skill when inserting them. I therefore sent two estimates to the other Aid organisation. I heard later that they had decided on the more costly option, no doubt because the local surgeon who was to be their medical consultant advised them to do so. He would be paid a standard monthly fee for his on-going support but his item of service payments would be almost non-existent if no IUDs were used.

I am aware that the IUD is a major plank in the family planning programmes of several countries. The reasons for this are complex and are often political as much as medical, more to do with prestige and image than with the needs of women who are rarely consulted before they are presented with a limited range of options, and among whom the phrase 'informed consent' has, in practice, no real meaning.

One Tuesday morning on our way to Hastings I was listening to the nurses chatting in Krio, as they usually did. I could follow most of what they said even when they were talking fast amongst themselves, but I was only listening with half an ear when I heard the word 'Logos'. This was no Krio term.

"What's Logos?" I asked.

"It's a boat," replied Zainah, "It comes every year in January and stays in the Port for a week."

"You can get books and it's very nice to see round it," added Jenneh who was one of the nursing team that week.

"Where exactly is it?"

"Oh, you know, it's in the docks, off Fourah Bay Road. You go down beside that secondary school. It's some sort of Christian ship. You should go, you'd find it interesting."

Fortunately the following Friday was not the last in the month so there was no staff meeting to hurry us back to Adelaide Street when the Kissy clinic was over and a visit to the Logos was hardly out of my way. Fourah Bay Road ran parallel with the notorious Kissy Road, but was even worse. It was nearer the sea and as it approached the city centre turned into Guard Street, which would easily have won the prize for the worst place in Freetown in which to break down.

I drove carefully along Old Kissy Road, circumnavigated the hidden depths of the permanent pond at the junction with the connecting track onto the main road, sped thankfully along the better surface and kept seaward to the right at the Up-Gun roundabout. Within half a mile I was in the Port area and on the pot-holed, rutted and largely non-existent surface of Fourah Bay Road. There was a great clutter of people walking, standing, squatting along the sides of the street. In some places the pavement was still intact but for most of the distance it was only present in parts so that two or three huge paving slabs would be missing after a stretch of several yards and the sidewalk would come to an abrupt halt over the top of the open drain.

The road went through a street market with stalls selling mounds of oranges, leaves, cassava, sweet potatoes and much smaller collections of 'Irish' potatoes, marble sized tomatoes, chillies, peppers and little heaps of spices that I could not identify. The sellers of clothes, T-shirts, children's dresses, men's shirts, cotton skirts and blouses used the chain-link fence round the Port Authority enclave to display their wares on coat-hangers hooked into the mesh. I saw one man who appeared to have only two shirts to sell, each on a coat-hanger, one in either hand. There was also a lot of wheeled traffic, the ubiquitous old bangers that served as taxis, mini-buses or poda-podas, ancient trucks which frequently broke down blocking 50 percent of the highway and bringing the traffic in both directions to a complete halt. Weaving their way in this maelstrom were two-wheeled carts with long shafts, usually heavily laden, with one man in front acting as a dray horse and another behind pushing and levering the vehicle round and over the holes in the surface and the vehicles parked haphazardly along the road.

I reached the turn off to the deep-water dock with relief. There were hardly any other vehicles down here and the road was quiet and, at first, shaded with trees. I was not certain that I had found the right turning, as I could not see the sea, let alone a ship, but in due course it curved round and there, moored alongside the dock, was a beautiful white ship. Without doubt, this must be the Logos. There were only three other cars parked on the quay side but there were several people walking over to the covered gang plank which attached the vessel to the shore. A good-looking, fair, bronzed young man was welcoming the visitors.

"Hi, folks, it's good to see you. Just walk right on up there and make yourselves at home but don't go anywhere outside the public decks please." He waved us into the relative darkness of what, in cruise ships, might be called the promenade deck. The open sides were closed by canvas awnings extending from the deck above to the bottom of the protective railings. These enclosed an extensive area from amidships to the stern. This was artificially lit and air-conditioned and was blissfully cool after the heat and humidity of the post-midday sun on the concrete dock outside. Open book stands were ranged along the perimeter of the space and more were arranged in islands away from the walls. Most of the books were paperbacks, many rewritten classics for both adults and children. Among a haphazard collection of cheap fiction I saw, to my astonishment, two books by the Australian writer of detective fiction, Arthur Upfield, featuring his half-caste policemen, Boney. I had a large collection of his works at home but he has been dead for some time now and most are out of print in the UK. I had not read either of these and picked them off the shelf with cries of jubilation loud enough to cause several people to look at me rather strangely. It was impossible to buy any books in Freetown except a very limited list of classic fiction used in the secondary schools and the English course at Fourah Bay College, so these were a real find. Although many of the books were cheap by Western standards, they were beyond the pockets of most of the locals, even school teachers and nurses, but the sale of books was not the main point of the exercise.

The Logos was a floating conversion factory manned by beautiful young people from wealthy backgrounds, largely American, who, from the highest motives, were cruising round the poorer ports of the world bent on saving the souls of the natives. The greater part of the books for sale were biblical with a strong evangelical flavour. At strategic intervals there was a beautiful young person of either sex, stationed to encourage the browsers to talk and ask questions. All the young evangelists I saw were good to look at, the men dressed in smart shorts and short sleeved shirts and the girls in skirts and blouses without any undue display of nubile flesh. They were all white skinned, the epitome of WASPs except one young man who was as black as his audience. I had bought a 'Sprite' to drink and was eating a doughnut from a small kiosk on the upper deck after I had been through the check-out from the book store. I was sitting on a bench with my back to an informal group of men who were gathered round the speaker. He certainly had their attention and was expounding a passage from the *New Testament*.

"Jesus said, Come unto me all you that labour. . . " It was a telling text and he spoke fluently and passionately. I have no doubt some of his audience would be greatly influenced and one or two perhaps even converted. To me there was something inherently distasteful about these well-heeled young people, whose shorts alone probably cost what most Sierra-Leonians had to live on for a month, coming here in an air-conditioned ship with all the trappings of Western living, talking to these Africans about saving their souls. At least the missionaries of an older generation lived with the people and many gave much of their lives in service to them, teaching or providing health care, as indeed some still do. I think they were misguided in many of their attitudes and practices but they were trying to put their Master's words into practical effect at considerable cost to themselves. The extreme Evangelical view that the saving of souls, by which is meant conversion by the equivalent of a sudden blinding flash on the way to Damascus, is the prime task of all those who truly follow the Lord, seems to me to be arrogant nonsense especially in the face of the poverty and destitution of most of Africa. These young people and their mentors were spiritual scalp hunters, bathing in the holy glow of knowing they were doing God's will and enjoying the delights of a tropical cruise at the same time.

As I drove back along Guard Street I made sure the windows were tightly closed and doors locked on the inside. This was partly to keep out the all pervading stench of sewage and rotting flesh from the corpses of dead dogs, cats and rats caught in the drains which, now there were no more rains to flush them out to sea, tended to get trapped below the sidewalks. The other reason was that thieves took advantage of any opportunity to relieve one of portable possessions. On my first drive through Guard Street with the off-side window half down, I had been almost stationary in the queue of traffic when a man shouted to me, "Missus, Missus, Yoh tiah be done flat."

I was concerned but I still had enough wit to remember that this was a common ploy used to distract one's attention and I was in time to see a brown arm snake in through the passenger side window. The fingers were grasping the handle of my battered old canvas briefcase but I was quick enough to lean across and wind up the window, trapping the errant limb. The thief immediately abandoned the attempt and his arm slipped out as serpent-like as it had slipped in. After that I had always kept my windows closed when I was in that end of the town, however hot it was.

Leona had experienced a much more unpleasant episode. She was being driven in a big four-wheel-drive vehicle and thought she was high enough up to risk having the window half open. She had had a small gold crucifix and chain brutally snatched off her neck. It was not of great intrinsic worth but had been given her in special circumstances which made it particularly valuable to her. She was not injured, apart from an unpleasant bruise round the back of her neck, but the incident shook her up more than she acknowledged at the time. In spite of these occurrences there was little threat of violence and I never felt in personal danger except from the traffic on the roads.

I was listening to the chest of a plump little pikin who was sitting on his mother's knee in the Main clinic about 11 o'clock one busy Monday, his T-shirt held up to his neck while I held my stethoscope against his back. His loose cough made it obvious that he had an infection but his mother was more likely to follow my instructions if she felt she had had her moneys' worth from the doctor. Using a stethoscope was part of the mystique.

"Mamie, he is a very fine child. You feed him good. I give you medicine for his cough and syrup for sleeping. . . " I was about to explain in more detail when Lauretta came round the curtain.

"Doctor Wilson, I'm sure you like to see this," and she beckoned me to follow. Excusing myself to my patient I went out into the narrow passage where minor procedures and injections were given. A handsome well built lady was standing with her back to me and her left side leaning towards the rather small window which afforded all the light there was in this part of the clinic. Sister Cline was about to open a boil on her shoulder which had come to a head. It was an unusual site for an infected lesion but it was not more than three-quarters of an inch across and I silently wondered why I had been invited to watch the proceedings.

Sister took a sterile needle and deftly decapitated the lesion. As the top came off a blind white maggot waved its head out of the central cavity, like a snake emerging from its egg. It was quite repulsive. With an exclamation of triumph Sister caught hold of it with a pair of forceps and drew it out of its human incubator, dropped it into the sink and squashed it with the bottom of one of the small bowls we used for holding swabs.

"A tumbu fly larva," she explained. "Haven't you seen one before?"

"No, I have not, and I'm not sure I want to again. What are they and where do they come from?"

"Tumbu flies lay their eggs on the lower leaves of trees and bushes, then when you walk under them or brush against them the grubs transfer to your clothing. They're so small you don't feel them burrowing into your skin and the first you know of it is when you get one of these lumps coming up. They're not really painful and you must not try to get them out before they are ripe, otherwise you leave some of the grub behind and it gets infected and you can have a nasty abscess. I'm sure if this woman's lesion had not been on her back, she would have dealt with it herself."

The following Thursday I was telling Carol this story at the golf club. She was very unimpressed.

"A friend of mine's husband had been camping up-country and had spread his shirt to dry overnight on some nearby bushes. A week or two later, I can't remember exactly how long, his back was covered in these tumbu boils. I can see her now on the beach at Tokay picking them out, fifty seven of them! There was hardly any normal skin to be seen! Of course," she added, "That's why it's essential to have one's clothes ironed, especially if they are hung outside to dry. The heat of the iron kills the grubs."

I had been hanging out my clothes under the trees since the rains stopped weeks before, and I had no practical access to an iron. After that I went back to drying my garments in the passageway, as I had done when it was wet. It was more than a month before I stopped wondering whether every little prickle and itch on my back might not be incubating a tumbu fly.

Chapter 7 – February
Unexpected Always Happen

THE MARIE-STOPES SOCIETY OF
Sierra-Leone had been negotiating with the Board of Management of
the Mission hospital at Segbwema to open a family planning clinic in
their premises. I did not know whether this was Sylvia's own idea or
whether she was being pushed by either the parent organisation in
London or by the Ministry of Health in Freetown or possibly both. All
our projects were in or around the capital, in nine different locations
but I knew that prestige was associated with activities 'Up-Line'.
Segbwema was only about two hundred miles away but because of the
appalling state of the roads it was a whole day's journey.

My personal view was that to extend our slender resources on such a
tenuous exercise was unwise, to say the least. Staff from Freetown who
could be trusted would have to be seconded on a rotating basis and live
there for three months at a time. The only vehicle that was capable of
surviving the murderous road was the old Land-Rover which frequently
broke down even in the city. There was no telephone that worked
connecting Segbwema with the outside world. In practice the two girls
working there would be on their own with no recourse to senior
management whether the problem was dishonesty or danger, but I could
see the attractions.

There had been a family planning clinic in the hospital until the
previous October. This had been funded by another Aid agency whose
financial support came from the USA. When President Bush, in his
wisdom, decided to withdraw federal funding from all contraceptive
organisations that were not opposed to abortion he condemned millions
of women world-wide, especially the poorest, to the tyranny of unrestrained fertility. It is probable that the abortion rate actually rose as,
once people have experienced the benefits of the higher standard of living
that is consequent on even a modest restriction in the number of off-
spring, they are prepared to go to considerable lengths to maintain it.

135

I pictured the many hundreds, possibly thousands of women, as I thought, who had been able to enjoy the benefits of a local family planning clinic for the past eight years and who had probably now become unpropitiously pregnant. There would be trained staff available on the spot in addition to our two headquarters staff, there was hospital back-up for medical problems and there was a lot of equipment, including six little motor-bikes for the use of the field motivators we would be sending out to the villages if the head-men agreed. Although in principle I thought the project misguided, in practice I was excited at the thought of the trip up-country and the three day break from the Freetown routine. I had never been farther from the city than Waterloo which was only twenty miles out.

The previous organisation had used hospital staff and administrators to run the daily clinics but Sylvia decided that it would be impossible to control the project unless we were completely independent. She had therefore negotiated to lease the premises from the hospital and rent accommodation for the Marie-Stopes staff who would be resident. The hospital engineers department who would be paid to carry out any necessary alterations and the doctor who would act as consultant would be paid a personal retainer. We would appoint our own staff, from the sister in charge to the field educators. These jobs had been advertised locally and our trip was to interview and select those we thought most suitable. We were to spend the night in Kenema, a town thirty miles or so beyond Bo, and travel the remaining twenty five miles to Segbwema the following morning.

An 'early start' had been planned ie 9am, and I was to be picked up by Sylvia on her way in to Adelaide Street where we were to meet the other members of our party. There were the usual inevitable delays and it was 10.30 before we were all sitting in the old Land-Rover. Sylvia, Sister Cline, Doctor (PhD) Joan, the Deputy Director and two other members of staff and, of course the driver. I had cherished an unspoken fantasy that we might have been going to travel in the new Peugeot estate car but was not surprised to find myself in my usual seat behind the driver which I occupied on our weekly trips to Hastings, Grafton and Jui. One had to sit slightly sideways as the distance between the back of the seat in front and the front of the seat behind was insufficient to accommodate the femoral length of even a woman of average height. This meant that first one buttock and then the other had to take priority on the seat and one either cold-shouldered one's immediate neighbour or was unable to enjoy an unimpeded view of the passing scene. Another minor discomfort was that the plastic upholstery of the seat squabs had become torn and damaged and you became increasingly aware of prickings and scratchings.

Soon after we passed Waterloo we drove for several miles between rows of gaunt palms, all dead or dying and the rusting remains of a considerable industrial plant beside the road. This plantation had been established to give productive employment to the prisoners in a penal settlement who had planted, tended and eventually harvested the nuts from the palm trees which were then crushed and the oil extracted. I never found out exactly what had allowed the project and the palm trees to die but the sight of acres of wasted effort returning to the bush seemed to typify so much of what was happening in the country and induced a mood of melancholy introspection. This was only broken when we stopped at Moyamba Junction and bought some sweet and juicy oranges from a strikingly attractive and cheerful girl at the roadside market. This was so typical of Sierra-Leone, just as one was thinking that there was really no hope, some contact with one of the people, cheerful, friendly and basically optimistic meant that one could not despair for long.

The road from Waterloo to the Port Loko turn-off was pock-marked with pot-holes like the face of a severe case of smallpox. However skilful the driver it was impossible to avoid them and, unless the crater was exceptionally wide, we drove on regardless, the passengers bouncing and lurching about, thrown first to one side and then the other, occasionally bouncing so hard that our heads hit the roof. Not surprisingly it was not long before the window on my side fell in, hitting my thigh with quite a thump.

The road from the Sixtieth Milestone to Bo was much better and consequently the noise inside the rattling old Rover was reduced enough for us to talk. The scrub along the roadside was dry and brown but although it had been cleared and burnt off along the edge, it presented an almost unbroken wall of small trees, saplings and cane grass over eight feet high in most parts. Every few miles we would drive through a village of small houses made of mud bricks or concrete and roofed with corrugated iron or thatched with palm. They were all tidy and clean and had none of the cast-off detritus of more affluent societies. There was no litter because there was nothing that was thrown away. Paper was precious, every bottle and container was used and used again. Nobody could afford cans of coke (the local version was bottled locally in Freetown) and 'take-away' food from street vendors was wrapped in leaves.

It was obvious that the earth was very fertile here and each village had patches of cultivation round it, growing bright green 'leaves' (rather like spinach and much used in so-called sauces) sweet potatoes, cassava and other vegetables. Rivers and streams provided fish, and small scrawny hens and sleek well fed goats wandered over the road and around the huts. I knew that rice was the staple item of the local diet and that Sierra-Leone had grown sufficient to feed its own people until three or four years ago. Since then the population had grown and the standards of husbandry had fallen and the cost of importing rice had become a major drain on the country's non-existent economy.

At intervals there were notices announcing an agricultural project sponsored by an Aid agency. Many of these were faded and far from new and some pointed down rough tracks away from the main road. The only piece of viable commercial agriculture I observed between Freetown and Bo was a small pineapple plantation which looked well tended and flourishing. The main road to Kenema bypassed Bo and we eventually reached the rest-house about 6 o'clock. Sylvia's husband was the manager of the bank in Kenema and the guest-house was in the same compound as his official residence. The compound was a little way out of the town in a slightly hilly, gently wooded area. There was a light breeze and the garden round the houses was laid out with well kept grass and flowering shrubs. Altogether it was a very welcoming haven after the discomforts of the day.

The next day it took an hour and a half to travel the twenty five miles to Segbwema. The road was so bad that we drove most of the time in four-wheel drive and never faster than twenty miles an hour, and this was the dry season. We crawled down the sides of huge pits and some how scrabbled our way out on the other side, we lurched from one promising set of parallel ridges into precipitous gullies when the ridges petered out without warning and all too literally let us down. We juddered over two miles of corrugated iron-hard clay and arrived nearly an hour late at 10.15am. The hospital was sited on a raised plateau to the south of the town, the single storey buildings scattered over a wide area with plenty of trees and natural foliage. We were greeted by a fat oily man in his early thirties.

"Welcome to the Methodist Mission Hospital," he said. "I have arranged everything for you." He went on to explain in detail.

"Of course many of the staff who were employed before have applied and I have given them my personal references. I was the director of the last family planning project and know the situation very well."

While he was talking he was ushering us along a concrete path beside a substantial building that stood on its own. He opened the door and indicated a table with several chairs behind it on the far side of the large room.

"I can give you a lot of help as I am sure you understand."

"Thank you very much for all your help, it was very good of you," replied Sylvia. "But there is no need for us to take up any more of your valuable time." She was gently but firmly ushering him to the door, and once there she shut it firmly with Mr Nyamba on the outside.

"I'm afraid you've made an enemy there," I commented. "He was mighty put out in every sense of the word."

"It's very important that we establish ourselves as completely independent from the hospital staff and especially the previous clinic."

How right she was became increasingly apparent as the day wore on. The most important post was that of the sister in charge and naturally the nurse who had previously held the job was one of the first to be interviewed. She had a fulsome testimonial from our friend Mr Nyamba and obviously expected to be appointed without delay. She spoke slowly and showed none of the enthusiasm that was so characteristic of our Marie-Stopes staff.

"Would you show us the register of patients and perhaps some of the clients' clinical notes?" asked Sister Cline.

"Oh, I can't do that we haven't got them anymore," she replied after some hesitation.

"About how many women did you see in a session?" I asked.

"I guess about ten or twelve on Fridays. That's market day in Segbwema and the people come in from the villages."

"What about the other days?" I persisted.

"Well perhaps there might be five or six."

We all realised that there had been only a minimal family planning service for many years but the director, the sister and the two or three other nursing staff had been collecting their salaries for doing very little while the field workers, we discovered later in the day, had been paid such a ludicrously small sum, even by local standards, that they had virtually given up.

It became apparent from the remarks of some of the other staff who had applied for their old jobs that the oily Mr Nyamba had assumed that he would again be the director. His unholy alliance with the surgeon who acted as consultant gynaecologist to the project would enable them to continue to line their pockets albeit that the funds would be coming from a different source.

The greatest number of vacancies and the largest number of applicants were for field workers to go out into the villages and motivate the people to use the family planning service. No previous experience was demanded but the person had to be literate and be able to understand and to a certain extent be able to converse in English, to speak Krio as well as their own native language and, most importantly, identify with the aims of the project.

There were more than twenty applicants for the six jobs and it was already 2 o'clock. We decided to divide them into four groups of five or six. There was only one man, a teacher who was very interested in community drama. He not only had better paper qualifications that the rest but his application form was well written and properly put together and was concise and pertinent to the post. He proved to be intelligent, lively, and with a deep commitment to the well-being of his country which he had already realised depended a great deal on controlling the growth of its tidal wave of people. Although he had had no previous experience in the contraceptive field, we unanimously decided to appoint him as field co-ordinator in the project. The other candidates were all young women who had completed their secondary education but were far from uniform in their abilities.

Having refreshed our minds with a further glance at their CVs we invited the first five to come in. Their looks and deportment belied their written forms. Here were attractive, sensible young women, not too overawed by being interviewed by five strangers and quite prepared to give their own views or undertake a role-play when asked to do so. By the time we had seen them all, it was obvious that it was going to be difficult to select the best. It was already nearly 5 o'clock and Sylvia was late for a meeting with the Paramount Chief, indeed she was so late that he had gone home leaving his deputy to accept her heartfelt apologies. The Land-Rover had then to take him, and a very ancient but extremely venerable lady whose role I never fathomed as she never spoke, back to their villages. We took the opportunity to inspect our prospective premises which we were going to lease from the hospital. These were the rooms which had been occupied (even if sparsely) by the previous organisation. We were going to buy most of the equipment that remained which included a generator and six little red motor-bikes for the field-workers. Fortunately we had not paid for these items, as, when the team returned two weeks later (without me on this occasion), they had all disappeared. Sylvia was told that they were the personal property of the surgeon/gynaecologist who had been the consultant to the previous clinic. He was subsequently suspended, I heard, for 'professional misconduct', ie being discovered *in flagrante delicto* with a student nurse. In a Methodist Mission hospital, financial irregularities could be overlooked but sins of a sexual nature were serious and could result in dismissal.

It was dark when we finally left the hospital and set out along the terrible road to Kenema. As the headlights lit up the convolutions and chasms of the track I was looking for a glimpse of monkey, deer, bird or snake taking a nocturnal outing from the bush on either side but I saw no more at night than I had during daylight. I fear that little is left of the formerly abundant wild-life since the native forests have been felled. Back in the rest-house we still had some homework to do, assessing the applicants and making final decisions before the impressions and appearances of each became blurred in our minds. After a welcome and satisfying evening meal I almost fell into bed by 9.30 in the only room fitted with an air-conditioner, powered by the bank's generator, and fell quickly asleep.

I was amazed to be offered Kellogg's conflakes for breakfast. Truth was I preferred toast as I did not really fancy them with powdered milk. I was glad to see that three of the others regarded the cereal as a real treat as I was afraid Sylvia had acquired them specially for me. She then carefully cut out a bit from the back of the packet and gave me the 'Family Rail' coupon (only valid in the UK). Even if it had been useable overseas the poor Sierra-Leoneans would have had to go to China to benefit as their only passenger railway had been sold, track, sleepers and rolling stock, to the Chinese eight years before. It delighted me to remember, when I was back in Scotland on leave, that my daughter's visit to me with my grandchildren had been facilitated by the thoughtfulness of another mother in West Africa who was brought up, as I had been, 'that nothing be lost'.

In spite of plans the night before for an early start back to Freetown, it was nearly 10.00am before we set off and it was soon apparent that our journey would be a long one. We were barely out of Kenema when the driver pulled up.

"I think we are losing water, the temperature is getting high." Sylvia had chosen the most reliable and competent of the three drivers and his diagnosis proved correct. We had to stop about once an hour to fill the radiator at village taps along our route. We also topped up with petrol on the rare occasions when there was a pump which was working, as it was usually only possible to buy four or five gallons at a time. Our fill-up at

Kenema had been possible because of our connection with the bank manager. Once past Bo we were on the bad road, our speed dropped, the water and petrol consumption rose and the noise and jolting became matters for endurance. We stopped at a small village market to buy some cassava for which the district was well known.

Sylvia then announced, "We might as well go and visit Port Loko while we are on our way home, it's not very far off our route and shouldn't take more than an hour or so."

Not very far! The turn off was about fifty miles from Freetown and a further forty miles, down a poorly surfaced road, was Port Loko. We were going to have to endure a further eighty miles on to our journey, at least three hours if I knew my Africans. It was three in the afternoon before we reached the fork and I had to abandon my ill-founded hope that Sylvia might change her mind as we were so late. The driver swung the old vehicle off the 'main' road and on we went. We came into a flat swampy landscape and eventually crossed the now unused small gauge railway that had carried iron ore from the mines at Lunsar to the abandoned deep water terminal at Pepil. We drove into Old Port Loko's single street and drew up outside a shabby but intact double-fronted bungalow.

We all got out and thankfully stretched our cramped limbs. No-one was in sight and Sylvia was clearly expecting to meet somebody. This was the man with whom she had been negotiating the buying of the house. She also hoped to see a man who could start on the repairs and alterations that would be needed. She sent the driver off to find these gentlemen after admitting that we were two hours later than she had expected. Even intelligent and experienced Africans have a very poor judgement of time!

Fortunately the driver returned quickly with a key and the promise of the imminent arrival of the owner. The key was what was really needed as Sylvia wanted our ideas on how the premises could be altered to make the best use of the rooms, especially as it was planned to be able to hold a weekly abortion session, when a doctor would come up from Freetown. Two nurses would also be in residence as it was too far for staff to travel daily.

I was much more whole-hearted in my enthusiasm for the Port Loko project than I was for that at Segbwema, principally because it was so much nearer the Marie-Stopes base in Freetown. Even so, the lack of mail and telephone services and the bad state of most of the road meant that it was going to be logistically difficult to keep in touch with the staff and maintain supplies. I had expressed my serious doubts about the financial viability and the problems of supervising the staff at Segbwema before I had even been there but she assured me that Marie-Stopes International in London were in favour of it and that so were the Government's Ministry of Health. She herself loved a challenge. The die was cast and I said no more.

By the time we reached the outskirts of Freetown it was completely dark and we were having to fill up with water every thirty minutes. As soon as we came into Kissy Road we knew there was trouble ahead. An almost stationary line of traffic snaked in both directions and only moved forward a yard or so at a time. It took twenty minutes to travel from number 169 Kissy Road to number 153, we crawled past at least three vehicles whose bonnets were up to allow easier egress for the belching clouds of steam caught in the lights of the headlamps.

We reached Adelaide Street at last, at 8.15pm. I was tired and stiff but glad to exchange the discomforts of the old Land-Rover for the upholstered quiet of my Ford Fiesta. I was home in fifteen minutes and even the difficulties of opening a tin of sardines by candle-light (which was not so dim that I could not fail to see that the ants had managed to get inside the tin in which I had stored a very stale roll of bread) could not dispel the pleasures of eating an insect enhanced sandwich after a long cold shower, and then lying stretched out on my bed in the dark listening to *The Forsyte Saga* on tape.

The next weekend I spent with Donald and Jane MacLeod and went straight to the main clinic on Monday morning. I was busy with their usual crowd of patient women, sickly babies and hypochondriacal youths from the Islamic Study Centre up the road. I was explaining to Mohomet, aged seventeen years, that the kick he had sustained from a fellow footballer's gym shoe had only caused minimal bruising and that he did not need to go for an X-ray. His face fell, but brightened when I added that perhaps he would feel better if a bandage were applied? Modified rapture. I heard a mutter.

"Chook? My body is weak, doctor." I gave up. "Very well, you can have your B Co injection."

"Thank you, Doctor." He jumped to his feet, no sign of the conspicuous limp with which he had entered the consulting room, and holding his prescription firmly in his hand, he went out to get his magic 'chook'. Many of these boys came from villages up-country and had never been away from their families and communities before. It was no wonder some sought a little personal attention, especially if it was marked by a bandage and accompanied by an injection.

At this point there were sounds of some major interruption above the general hub-bub and Sister Cline came round the curtain.

"I think you'd better come Doctor. Mrs King has come from Adelaide Street. There has been a break-in at your flat."

Apparently Mrs Brown, my landlord's wife, had telephoned the office when Musu, the daytime watchman, had noticed that the air-conditioner was missing from my flat, leaving a large rectangular hole in the wall about five feet up from the ground. Although this had been discovered about 9 o'clock the vagaries of the telephone system had meant that, although Mrs Brown's phone was working, that in the main clinic only a mile down the same street, was not. So Sylvia had had to come herself, as soon as she and a vehicle with a driver were free.

My immediate reaction to the news was a gut-wrenching thought. Passport, money, camera, radio, tape recorder would probably all have gone, and the absence of the last two would seriously affect my ability to adjust to the lack of power, especially during the twelve nightly hours of darkness. They could not be replaced until I went home on leave, another two months hence. However, this was speculation, the important thing was to go home and inspect the damage for myself.

I drove back with Sylvia and we were greeted by a distressed Mrs Brown. We gazed at the empty space and the black scuffing of toes near the bottom of the wall. I unlocked the padlock on the door and went in. Everything looked the same in the hall. I went into the bed-sitting room. As usual the wardrobe doors hung open. I never closed them because of the risk of mildew, the small bookcase was in its normal position alongside my bed with its closed back to the window. It was on these shelves that I kept all the items I most valued, including money and passport, radio and tape recorder. They were all there, untouched and it was evident that the thieves had not actually entered the flat. It was a huge relief not only to me, but also to my boss and my landlady.

The latter had already called the police and three uniformed men were waiting to take a statement from me. They were obviously disappointed when they realised that it was only the air-conditioner that had gone.

"We need dash to buy paper and pencil to write statement," the older-looking man said.

"I will give you paper and lend you a pencil," I replied, much to their obvious dismay. I duly provided them with what was necessary and my simple account was laboriously written down. I said I had been away for the weekend and the air-conditioner had been there when I left. Nothing else had been stolen. Then, rather mischievously I said, "What about these beautiful finger-prints on the wall?"

For there were the clear imprints of four fingers from each hand on the clean white paint where somebody had pulled himself up by his fingers to look through the gap, once the air-conditioner had been taken out.

"But I don't suppose you have a finger-print expert in Sierra-Leone do you?" I asked innocently.

"Oh yes, Missus, we have finger-print officer. You pay dash and he will come."

"You mean I would have to pay?" I asked in pretended astonishment. "I don't think I'll bother, all the same."

The last thing I wanted was for the thief to be caught. I had heard too many awful stories of people who had got entangled in the web of justice. In particular that of a Dutchman who had had some small item of value, his watch I think, snatched from him when he was driving through Kissy Street. Unfortunately for him a bystander gave chase and the man was eventually caught and charged. The Dutchman worked for an Aid agency and his term of service was due to expire about three months later. He was, of course, a material witness and was informed that he could not be granted an exit visa until the case was heard. His departure was delayed four months and, so I was informed, involved considerable outlay to the officials in charge to encourage them to expedite the matter. In the end he was allowed to make a sworn statement accompanied by a handsome gift to the forces of law and order and was then permitted to depart.

There was little doubt that my air-conditioner had been stolen by the night watchmen, of whom there were three. One, a cheerful rascal known as Soloman, I had treated for a large chronic tropical ulcer on his shin. Three times a week for six weeks I had cleaned, swabbed and dressed it, before it healed. This, at no cost to him, and in my own time, at night and at weekends. It had not prevented him sometimes from clutching his stomach in assumed agony, due to imaginary hunger pains, when he opened the compound gates for me after I had been out for the evening, and asking for a 'dash' to buy rice. As he was an exceptionally fit young man and far from emaciated, I greeted these requests as a joke, occasionally asking him if he wanted the 'dash' deducted from the regular weekly payment I gave to him and his fellow guards. He was unwilling to agree to this but once or twice I had given him a small sum to go and buy beer, as I knew that this was what all his play-acting was about. So, to some extent we understood one another. Perhaps these things had something to do with why no-one had actually gone into the flat and robbed me but, more probably, they had been interrupted and given up. I will never know.

Their story was graphic. They had heard the thief and tried to catch him but he had run away up the side of the bungalow and scrambled over the six foot thorn hedge, managing to kick off Soloman's attempt to hold on to his foot. I inspected the scene of his courageous intervention, where not a twig was broken, not a leaf disturbed.

"That was very brave of you, Soloman. He must have been an exceptionally tall strong man to carry that heavy air-conditioner under his arm and climb this hedge. I am very grateful to you for trying, but unfortunately, as you did not manage to catch him or get the air-conditioner back, I am afraid I cannot give you a dash."

He gave me a half smile and almost said aloud, "It was worth a try anyway," and he would not have been referring to the fictional attempt to apprehend the thief. Later on in my stay in Sierra-Leone he tried to repeat the tactic of being rewarded for rectifying a situation which he and his cronies had created. I was going to bed one night when there was a hammering on my kitchen window. Considerably annoyed I opened the casement.

"Please, Doctor Wilson your car is not locked. Give us the key and we will lock it for you, then perhaps you will give us a dash?"

It so happened that I knew the car was properly locked up as I had had a particular reason to check it. It was after I had injured my shoulder and it was the first day of my African driver. He and I had meticulously checked both doors before he had gone home. On any other night I might not have been so positive, although it was such a vital precaution that I do not think I had ever forgotten.

"In that case, I think I had better come and check it myself."

This produced the expected protests. They had no doubt waited until they thought I was undressed and in bed. It was not only that I had no intention of handing over a reward for an imaginary good deed but the risk of an impression of the key being taken while it was out of my possession was a very real one. I hitched up my nightie and put on a skirt and blouse on top, unbarred the inner door, unlocked the padlock on the outside one and stepped outside, re-padlocking it behind me. I was escorted by the two men to the upper compound to inspect the Fiesta.

As I had known would be the case, it was still safely locked. Abu Kamora protested that on his word as a policeman (which was his day time occupation) the car had been unlocked when he tried it. "It must have been a Juju that relocked it then." I said and retired once more to bed.

When I was a passenger in the Marie-Stopes Land-Rover on our weekly trips to Jui, Grafton and Hastings I was able to observe many fascinating and intriguing aspects of the streets that passed me by when I had to concentrate on my driving. The names of the roads – Priscilla Street, Annie Walsh Lane, Rawdon Street, Wellington Street, Bathurst Street and so on reflected the founding of the first British colony in Africa in 1806. The freed slaves themselves who formed the nucleus of the population of Freetown bore English and Scottish names and still do, to this day. There is a 'Nicol' Lane in the city and one of the Marie-Stopes nurses was called Rebecca Nicol which (with an extra 'l') had been my own name before I was married. The Fraser family have a long and distinguished history of service to their country but are totally African. To an outsider the name of the eminent gynaecologist with an Aberdeen medical degree, Doctor George Bernard Fraser might conjure up an image of an expatriate Scot, but he is a native Sierra-Leonian and proud of it. There are other street names which reflect more recent history, Siako Stevens Street (a former president) and OAU Drive, a memorial to the disastrous visit of the Organisation of African Unity in 1982 which effectively bankrupted the country.

Many of the clapped out old bangers which served as taxis, the ancient minibuses known as poda-podas, which provided a very sketchy and unreliable form of public transport, especially from the outlying and up-country districts, and the heavy trucks which were in such a bad state of repair that they were a constant menace to all other road users, were embellished with mottoes and phrases which were sometimes singularly appropriate. Many invoked the deity – 'God bless', 'God's time is best', 'I hope to God', 'Nar God dae gee' (only God gives). Others were more personal – 'Let them say' was very popular indicating the driver's defiance of the world. 'Let my enemies live long and see what I be in the future' was even stronger. Some were philosophical – 'There is a time for every proposal', 'Wan world', 'Be patient'. A few which I observed more than once, were completely inexplicable – 'Terror in Tokyo', 'No 1 the Burning Train'. Some displayed the humorous cynicism which I so much enjoyed in the Africans 'No money No woman', 'White teeth Black

147

heart'. I wrote them down in my little notebook and collected over fifty in two journeys to the outlying clinics.

On this Tuesday, towards the end of February, we were coming back into the city along the main road from the hinterland. The scrubby vegetation had been cut back from the road margins and burnt off, exposing dry, khaki coloured undergrowth and the baked red earth. In front of us an aged bus was grinding along, baskets piled high on the roof and the sides festooned with passengers unable to squeeze inside and forced to cling to window and door frames. It was grossly overloaded and thick black smoke was pouring from its exhaust. Our driver had made several attempts to pass it but the bus driver was not keen on this idea and by sticking to the middle of the road until on-coming traffic forced him over, he had succeeded in condemning us to several miles of carbon monoxide poisoning.

Suddenly the bus swerved violently but the driver miraculously managed to hold it on the tarmac as an off-side wheel shot across the road ahead of the vehicle and came to rest in the opposite ditch. The exposed metal of the axle scored the surface and produced a jet of sparks which set fire to what was left of the road-side vegetation. Even before it managed to stop the extraneous passengers were jumping off and several more somehow got out of the windows. No-one appeared to be hurt and we drove past without stopping but I had had time to remember, in the time when we were behind it, that it bore the message 'Unexpected always happen'.

I had been invited to go with friends to spend a weekend on a national nature reserve at Tiwai Island, in the Moa River. Jim was the manager of the Auriol Tobacco Company, and his wife Carol had her mother staying with them for a holiday. Ida was a remarkable lady, she had a natural spontaneity and warmth that bridged all the usual barriers between youth and age, black and white, with only a minimum of words in common. She was game for any experience and was equipped with a battery operated tape recorder and video camera.

We were to set out from their house on Friday morning but Carol had been smitten with a nasty attack of the runs. However, after resting for an hour or so, she gamely decided that the worst was over and, after a minor panic about adequate supplies of imodium, which I had fortunately brought with me, we set out in the very comfortable four-wheel drive Japanese vehicle, well upholstered and air-conditioned. The contrast with my trip in the old Land-Rover two weeks before, was marked and duly relished!

We were on the narrow unsurfaced road to Zimmi which is the main route to Liberia. Before long we saw an inconspicuous sign to Tiwai – this track was a definite improvement on its predecessor as the traffic was infrequent, with few heavy trucks. Eventually, as dusk was falling, we arrived at the village on the river bank from which we had to embark for Tiwai Island.

As soon as we drew up we were surrounded by a score of children of all ages eager to earn a dash by carrying our baggage down a rather steep, muddy path to the water's edge. The heaviest piece, the cold-box, containing beer, coke, 7-Up and so on for the four of us for two days, was lifted onto the head of a girl who judging by her relatively short stature and budding breasts was not more than twelve years old. My hold-all was grabbed by a wiry little boy who was about half that age. Ida and I followed, in as dignified a way as we could manage, clutching at branches, or even twigs, to help us keep on our feet as we skidded down to the river. We hid our dismay at the sight of our transport with admirable aplomb. Two dug-out canoes were resting with one end in the mud of the bank, they did not even appear to be tied up. The smaller was about six feet long and had a distinct lateral curve, rather like a banana. There was an inch or two of water in the bottom and no seats. This was soon rectified by a few quick chops with a machete on a convenient branch and the resultant batons were jammed across the bottom just clear of the puddle. The other canoe was much bigger but was already loaded amidships with two very large square packing cases full of provisions and equipment for the scientific and Peace-Corps worker's camp. These were accompanied by two girls who were taking the supplies back to their base.

While all these matters were being sorted out, Ida was busy communicating with the children. It was nearly dark but she propped herself against the roots of a tree and started to record them and then played the tape back. The children were wildly excited and within minutes were clapping rhythmically and singing, all of which she duly recorded. Ida and I were allocated to the small canoe as we were assessed, correctly, as not being agile enough to climb over the baggage in the larger one. When we were settled or, in my case more accurately, jammed in, our Mende paddler scrambled into the back and pushed off. I gripped the sides as we rocked alarmingly only to find the tips of my fingers were in the water! I remembered that we had been told that we would be very lucky to see a crocodile as they had nearly all been slaughtered for their skins. The memory remained, not very far back in my mind, until we were once more on dry land.

We crossed the brown swirling water and then were paddled downstream parallel with the island until, after twenty minutes, we were landed on another muddy bank. By this time it was dark, although still only 7pm but a walk of two or three hundred yards brought us to the camp. There was a central eating/relaxing area with a palm-thatched roof with open sides. A rectangular table and chairs occupied the half nearest the cook-house; round the central support were shelves containing a varied assortment of books of reference, maps of the reserve and helpful leaflets, all a bit tattered and mouldy but still usable. Hammocks hung from the roof beams in the rest of the space and the four sleeping tents were spaced round about. Of course, I did not take all this in at once, but had time to observe the arrangements after Ida and I had been shown our quarters. We were to share a strong nylon tent, zipped up the middle against mosquitoes, and thatch had been erected above it to give protection in the rains.

We were tired with the journey but Carol miraculously coaxed the wood cooking fire to life and produced hot tasty spaghetti bolognese in what seemed no time at all. We went to bed early, each tent held two beds – thin foam mattresses on slightly raised wooden platforms. We had brought our own sheets and pillows. Mine was the only one I had, a cheap cotton ticking overfilled with chunky lumps of plastic foam, impossible to bend or manipulate, and not very comfortable. I went to sleep fairly quickly and was woken at two in the morning by the sound of a shot. It sounded some distance away and I was just reassuring myself by remembering that poaching monkeys on the mainland was common practice as monkey meat was a much prized delicacy among the local tribes, when a second shot resounded through the night. This time I reminded myself that no Africans would spend the night on Tiwai because it was inhabited by bad spirits, and this was what had saved the chimpanzees and the other species of monkey from extinction. There was a brilliant moon and the cleared area of the camp shone with a white light reflected on the paths and walls of the tents. As usual by this time in the night, I felt the need to go to the loo but I was rather reluctant to venture out into that brilliant white light and walk the hundred yards to the little hut. At this moment a loud barking cry sounded from the nearby forest. I thought at first it was a man calling in anger to someone else, but it was not repeated and I realised it was probably a monkey. I was sufficiently in doubt to opt out of venturing out of my tent, however full

FEBRUARY

my bladder. Eventually after lying tensely under my sheet for some time I gradually relaxed and fell asleep.

The next morning we were free to roam where we liked along the grid of tracks in the Northern third of the Reserve, mapped and maintained by the Peace Corps volunteers. This was made available to tourists like us for a very modest sum. All water for drinking had to brought across to the island by boat and was carried in repeated journeys by bucket on the head of a particularly graceful African woman who tipped it into a large drum which was freshly filled each day.

Tiwai was especially known for the numerous species of monkey and the chimpanzees which still inhabited this last remnant of the rain-forest which, until recently, covered much of Sierra-Leone. The island is about five miles long and two and a half miles wide and a considerable amount of observation and research was being conducted in the Southern part which was rightly out of bounds to those not involved. Anglia Television were making a film about the wildlife and several very tall platforms had been built to bring observers and cameras level with the tree canopy.

We had arranged for a guide to take our party to the best locations to see the various types of monkey, but he was not available until after 3.00pm. So, map in hand, I strolled off to explore this fascinating new environment. There had been no rain for over three months and the ground was littered with crisp fallen leaves from the tropical evergreens in the tree tops hundreds of feet above, and the scrub and saplings, which grew wherever a patch of sunlight could reach the forest floor. I wandered happily for over two hours and, although I only identified one monkey (a green) I saw over sixteen different species of wonderful butterflies. I briefly noted down the most obvious characteristics, the often brilliant colours with fantastic patterns in browns or black on the undersides of the wings, the variety of wing shapes and the differences in size, from tiny white 'ghost' moths to purple and chestnut giants five inches across. I hoped to be able to identify them with the help of the reference books back at base but the one devoted to lepidoptera only had pictures of three that I could recognise. My pleasure at seeing these wonderful creatures was not really diminished by not being able to identify them but another part of me would have experienced considerable satisfaction if I had.

After a snack and drinks from the cold-box, which revived us all, we relaxed in the hammocks or lay on our beds until it was time to collect ourselves together for the afternoon's foray. The others had seen one colony of monkeys on their morning safari and the African guide started

151

us off in the same direction. He certainly knew their whereabouts but monkeys are extremely mobile. Fortunately most colonies are very noisy and advertise their presence in the tree tops by shouts and screams that can sound very human at a distance. Also they make a great commotion in the foliage as they follow their leader leaping from one slim branch to the next. However, they are not always on the move and the whole colony can be almost invisible from the ground except to the expert eye of the guide. It was hot and very humid and the going was rough, although I am sure he moderated his usual pace considerably, in view of our white hairs. Ida had an arthritic hip and managed along uncomplainingly but her limp became more noticeable and, after an hour or so, she decided to return to camp. Alan volunteered to go with her as we were quite a long way from base In spite of the grid map, it was difficult to find one's way when there were no long vistas or obvious landmarks to tyros like us.

Carol and I went on. She was carrying the video camera and we were able to view five different species of monkey, the black and red colobus being the most spectacular, perhaps because they were so active. After having the privilege of watching troops of these free-swinging exuberant creatures in their true environment how can one acquiesce in their confinement in a cage? But, this is the only place in Sierra-Leone where they can be seen in even limited numbers. Virtually all the rest have been eaten, not by rapacious Europeans but by hungry Africans.

We plodded on and my relief was great when we emerged on the far side of the island onto a wide sandy beach and the flowing waters of the Moa. As we crackled through the dry undergrowth onto the sand, a huge minotaur lizard moved with lightning speed round the half circumference of the beach. It must have been over six feet long and as thick as a small tree trunk. It was gone before Carol even had time to think of the camera, let alone position it. I plunged my feet, elastic stockings and all, into the cooling river, then reluctantly pushed them back into my shoes before heaving myself up for the long slog home. And it was a long slog. I had had virtually no exercise since I left Glasgow six months before. I had no stairs in my flat, did not walk to work and had never appreciated the joys of playing golf and here I was, trudging grimly in the footsteps of the guide though a tropical rain forest, having walked already for more than two hours with only a ten minute break to take my weight off my feet. Carol called back.

"How are you doing, Libby?"

"OK as long as we're going back now!"

It was nearly dark when we saw the lights of the camp glinting through

152

the trees. We had been on the move for three hours. Every bone, joint, and muscle in my body was screaming out for respite; the relief of sitting down was inexpressible. I was so tired that I could hardly remain upright long enough to eat. I was selfishly glad to realise that Carol had also found it quite an ordeal, but neither of us would have opted out, even if we had had the chance.

The next morning, when we were packing up to go, a girl from the Peace Corps camp arrived with mail she asked us to post in Freetown. She told us that a young Englishman who was finding his own way round West Africa, had bought a canoe in Kenema, a market town about thirty miles up-river and two nights later, when he was camped on the bank, it had been stolen back by the man who had sold it to him. The local villagers thought this was a great joke and the story had arrived with the fresh water supply that morning. We were soon on our way back across the Moa, only this time we were all in the same boat and our passage was both more dignified and less hazardous. Ida persuaded the Mende paddler to sing a traditional song as he stroked us along and she recorded it, which delighted him greatly when she played it back. It took a little time to get the baggage carried up and stored in our vehicle and we were able to wander about the village and observe what was going on. The people did not seem to mind our interested stares and a few could speak Krio. There was a central meeting house of thatched palm with open sides. There were no seats but about a dozen hammocks hung from the rafters. This was a 'men only' zone. Presumably the horizontal position increased the blood flow to the head and clarified the thought processes but I thought it would make a very comfortable venue for the sociable consumption of palm-wine and probably was the African equivalent of the local pub in England.

Two girls of about five and seven were winnowing some grain but I could not make out what; a man who had a good command of English was making a rope sling to be used to climb the trees to tap the palm wine and several groups of women were cooking on small fires of wood on the open ground between the palm thatched huts. As we were about to climb into the car a tall good-looking youth of eighteen or nineteen walked over and introduced himself in the unmistakable accent of an English public school. He was certainly travelling light, his rucksack was half collapsed on his back and onto it was tied a plastic bag containing some rather limp-looking plants. He told us of his misadventure with the canoe with great good humour, and said it had all been for the best as he had been forced to walk along the bank of the river, which had been botanically much more productive than lying in a boat while the current did all the work. As we drove back to relative civilisation I regretted very much that we had not thought to ask him for a name and telephone number we could have contacted in the UK, just to let somebody know that their son or brother was alive and flourishing especially if they had heard nothing for three months.

Two weeks later rebel forces from Charles Taylor's army in Liberia invaded Sierra-Leone and came up the Moa in their canoes. The Peace Corps camp, the research station and the Anglia film unit were all evacuated in a hurry. The rebels still control Tiwai and I fear they have no respect for local taboos but they are very fond of roast monkey.

Chapter 8 – March
I Bit Her Buttock Hard

ONE SATURDAY MORNING EARLY IN
March, I went up to Carol's about 10 o'clock to find out whether Ida was
planning to travel on the Hovercraft to catch the KLM plane from Lungi,
on which we were both travelling back to the UK. I was going home on
a months leave in mid-March, which was in about two weeks. When I
arrived at their house Carol said,
   "We're just about to go on a trip in Duncan's boat to Buntz Island.
Why don't you come too?"
   "But I hardly know Duncan, I can't just gate-crash his party!"
   "I know he won't mind, there's only Mum and I and Betty and one
more won't make any difference. We are taking a picnic and there's more
than enough for everyone." I did not take much more persuading; the
thought of a boat trip to the notorious Buntz Island which had been
used by the French for slave trading, instead of spending six hot and
humid hours in my flat, was an option that required no lengthy
deliberation and without even a pretence of demurring I joyfully accepted.
I left the Fiesta in their compound and we went down to the Aqua Sports
Club in Carol's four- wheel drive vehicle.
   Freetown is a succession of bays and inlets which have been used by
naval and merchant vessels for over two hundred years. Duncan was
unusual for an expatriate, in that he had lived in Sierra-Leone for eleven
years. His boat was his passion and his hobby and he knew the coast as
well as he knew the road from his house off Spur Road to his office in
the town centre.
   We rounded the promontory of Murray Town, crossed the inlet of
Whiteman's Bay and skirted the rounded knob of King Tom. I was
interested to see the Commonwealth War graveyard from a totally
different angle, and there was the clinic, behind the old naval cannons
still pointing out to sea. By this time we were in Kroo Bay where the
worst slums in the city spill on the sewage soaked mud into the water. I

was glad we were off-shore and could not smell the stench, but passing this visible reminder of the plight of so many, did subdue our holiday spirits for a time.

Soon we were crossing Destruction Bay and had to keep farther out, as we were approaching the deep water quays and rounding the headland into Cline Bay. As we moved along, our host pointed out the name and former history of each of the wrecks whose rusty superstructures were all too visible in the shallower water in-shore. It was a bit like a guided tour of the wall monuments in Westminster Abbey. There was hardly a space between them and they spanned a period of over sixty years. Presumably the ships that had ended their days in Freetown in an earlier era had eventually disintegrated to such a degree that they now lay so far below the surface that they could no longer be seen, even at low tide. Even so, we were shown the wrecks of three previous generations of ferries and we all agreed that the present vessel would probably be joining this melancholy sub-aqua club before long.

Once past Cline Bay it was time to stop hugging the shore and set course for our destination. We swung north into the estuary of the Sierra-Leone river which was here about seven miles across, and bisected the ferry crossing from the Lungi peninsula to the Kissy terminal in Freetown. The estuary is formed by the confluence of three wide creeks, the banks low lying and covered by mangrove swamps, the ideal breeding ground for mosquitoes and the reason for the epithet 'white man's grave'. The 'river' widens to nearly twice the width of its narrowest part as one goes up-stream. The numerous islands can hardly be distinguished from the 'main' land unless the navigator knows his way. We were running with the tide and the wind was behind us so we made good progress over a relatively calm sea.

After an hour or so I could see what appeared to be an enormous bridge on the northern shore, stretching from a relatively high promontory until it ended abruptly, more than a hundred yards into the water. As we moved nearer, it was possible to see that this was a huge conveyor belt and loading gantry. Duncan said that this was all that remained of the Sierra-Leone iron ore company. The crude ore had been extracted up-country near Lunsar and brought nearly a hundred miles by train on a specially constructed railway to this terminal, for removal by deep water ships. The railway is still marked on the map, the small gauge rails remain in situ, and this huge, virtually indestructible steel skeleton bears witness to man's ability to find solutions as long as the end result is profitable. But the total abandonment of the site, the desolation and the triumph of the mangrove forest also have a tale to tell.

It is a sight Europeans only see if they, like us, were travelling up-river to the slave island. Now the iron ore has stopped coming there is no longer any reason to stay in Pepel, the road is impassable, the railway defunct. Although arriving by boat is still possible, what is there to land for, anyway?

Soon we were able to identify Buntz, a small island only a mile and a half across, wooded, with some fine trees on the slightly raised central plateau, circled by a narrow band of green inside the encircling beach. The substantial remnants of stone buildings stood up among the vegetation. Fortunately, Carol had been here once before and was able to take us round the ruins. Duncan had elected to stay with his boat, but the rest of us walked up a well marked path onto a flat platform with a dozen or so cannon, mounted, and pointing out to sea. Each was stamped with the royal GRIII cipher. It was strange to place one's hand on one of these metal monsters and think that it had been hauled into place nearly two hundred years ago by press-ganged ordinary seamen from Plymouth and Portsmouth, who probably never lived to tell their tales back home.

We were about to explore the central quadrangle where the slaves were paraded. Here potential buyers could view them from above, without risking injury to health or person by too close contact with the wretched captives. We heard a shout and turned to see an elderly African hurrying towards us. He carried a rather battered old attaché case which he carefully placed at the roots of a tree. His dugout canoe was drawn up on the beach and it was evident that as soon as he had seen our boat approaching the island he had paddled across the mile or so of water in order to be our official guide. We were very willing to be guided and Carol was quite happy to relinquish her role, even if her recollections of what she had been told by the University historian on her last visit, did not completely coincide with his.

The gist was the same. The French were the baddies who established the settlement for the sole purpose of having a base to which the hi-jacked Africans could be brought and kept safely, with no chance of escape, until the Spanish and Portuguese slave merchants who transported them across the Atlantic, came to select their merchandise. The British, by means of an under-cover agent, succeeded in invading the island and throwing out the French, and it had remained under British sovereignty until independence in 1961. The old man's English was not very good and the more he talked the more he lapsed into Krio, but it was not difficult to follow most of his comments.

After a thorough exploration of the ruins, he led us along a fairly well marked path to the other end of the island. There, among several tall trees and surrounded by scrub was a small graveyard. There were half a dozen recognisable graves some of which had been deliberately vandalised, the table-top tomb stones broken by blows from an axe or a sledge hammer. Two or three were still standing, half buried in the earth, and the inscriptions were easy to read.

One marked the grave of a young woman whose father had been a sea-captain, and others were of military personnel who probably died, not of wounds, but of fever. Our guide lamented the day the British had left. He looked nostalgically back to the old colonial days when the island was a tourist attraction that merited a 'visitor's centre'. He showed us the almost totally disintegrated remains of a small round hut which, he assured us, had had a fine palm thatched roof and which had housed a table and chair where he himself sat to welcome visitors, before taking them on the guided tour. He spoke with pride of how the paths were properly cleared, the ruins prevented from further deterioration and the grass was cut, conjuring up a picture of some English castle lovingly cared for by the Ministry of Works. Indeed, it was probably exactly like that and no doubt provided regular employment for some of the men on the adjacent mainland. The present rough, but not ineffective clear up had been done by young volunteers from the Peace Corps or VSO.

The purpose of the attaché case then became apparent. He opened it almost reverently and took out a rather dog-eared black ledger. This was the visitor's book for Buntz Island. He produced a ball point pen with which we were to sign our names. There were pathetically few recorded in the past few years, a few groups of six or eight French names and places of origin – tourists brought by fast sea-launch from the luxury hotel at Tokay on the Freetown peninsula. I wondered if the old man was sophisticated enough to edit his history for his audience.

One morning at Adelaide Street a smart young woman came in and asked if she could buy some ampicillin capsules, Admiya, the receptionist, brought her in to see me.

"I have told her we do not sell drugs except to our patients and she must pay a consultation fee and see a doctor or nurse first, but she says she is not ill. . . "

It was nearly 1 o'clock and there were no more clients waiting.

"Come and sit down. Why do you want the antibiotic? Have you a problem you do not want to tell the clerk?" I thought she might be worried that she had contracted a venereal disease.

"Oh no Doctor, I am quite well. I want the ampicillin for my periods."

"What do you mean, your periods?"

"Well, I think it is good to make sure all the badness that goes out of my body every month is properly cleaned away and the ampicillin will take care of any germs that are left behind." She hesitated slightly, "The trouble is, that I don't think it is working as well as it used to."

"How long have you been taking the capsules?" I asked her.

"I started about a year ago. I don't take them all the time, only for the four or five days that my period lasts each month."

"What makes you think they are not working anymore?"

"It's just that I've felt really itchy down there for the last few weeks and, however much I wash, it always comes back. I'm sure it's nothing serious but I thought perhaps I should be taking the ampicillin all the time instead of just for a few days each month. Only it costs such a lot and I thought you might be cheaper than the chemist."

"Don't worry, Nadine, there are no germs in your womb at any time, and although the lining is shed each month when your period comes, this is not 'bad' blood which will make you ill if it stays inside. It is just nature's way of preparing your body for the arrival of the next egg into your womb in the next month. As you know, if the egg is fertilised by a sperm the tiny embryo attaches itself to the lining which helps it to grow, then it doesn't come away, you have no period, and you know you are pregnant."

For a moment she looked horrified and I realised I had gone a little too fast for her and that her command of English, or biology, was not as sophisticated as her appearance and occupation (secretary) suggested.

"No, no I don't mean you are pregnant, just that you are almost certainly perfectly healthy and there is no need for you to take an antibiotic every month. Suppose I give you a check up down there and put your mind at rest?"

She readily agreed to this and quickly climbed onto the couch with her pants off. I asked Keturah, the nurse on duty, to hold the torch so that I could have a good look at Regina's vulva. It was a little reddened and had whitish patches on the surface of the mucous membrane especially round the vaginal opening and in the crevices between the outer and inner lips. The appearance was typical of thrush, whose presence I had suspected ever since the girl had mentioned her itchiness. I gently examined her internally and was able to reassure her that, apart from the mild infection with thrush, she was very healthy in that part of her body and should have no problems having a baby when she wanted one. She got dressed and sat down at the table beside me.

"The reason you've got this thrush infection is because you've been taking the ampicillin. It sometimes happens after only one course and you've taken it for five days every month for nearly a year! Never mind, no real harm has been done. I will prescribe some special kind of tablets, called pessaries, which you put up inside your passage every night for a week, and that should cure it, as long as you don't take any more antibiotics!" I wrote a note on her case-card and then looked up,

"Do you want to have a baby just now?"

"Oh no, Doctor, I have a good job and I don't want to get married or have a child for at least a year," she paused, "but I do have a boy friend. I've been too frightened of getting pregnant to go with him very often and since I've had this itch I've been afraid to let him come near me, in case I gave him a germ."

"So you haven't used any family planning?" She shook her head. "Would you like to talk it over with Sister Cline?" I asked her. "She can tell you about all the different methods and you can decide which one would suit you best." Regina agreed to this with alacrity and Sister told me later that she had been happy to take the pill and had an appointment to return for further family planning in three months.

Vulval thrush was not the only condition I had observed when I examined her. She was the third female I had seen gynaecologically in Freetown who had an intact clitoris. The subject of female circumcision is a very emotive one and I had been made aware of the extent of this practice in Sierra-Leone well before I left the United Kingdom. I had been at an international symposium in Marrakesh in the preceding November and had been impressed by a strikingly good-looking African woman who was manning a small stand in the main concourse. She was handing out free leaflets and trying to sell a book she had both written and published, *The Circumcision of Women, A Strategy for Eradication*.

This was Doctor Olayinka Koso-Thomas. At that time I had no idea that nine months later I would be living in Sierra-Leone myself but, working as I did in the field of women's reproductive health, it was a subject in which I had been interested for a long time. About ten years before we had had a Sudanese woman doctor as a trainee for her Family Planning Certificate at the main teaching clinic at Claremont Terrace in Glasgow. She had felt so strongly about this mutilating custom that she had not only informed us of what was involved but had allowed the woman doctors working there at the time to see the result on her own body. I can still remember what I saw. Nothing horrendous in the way of scars or traumatised tissue, nothing deformed, there was nothing there at all, a smooth art of slightly shiny mucous membrane continuous with the inner lining of her labia majora; no clitoris, no labia minora; it was as though she had been born without these normal parts of female anatomy.

I talked to Dr Koso-Thomas for some time and discovered that when she had written her book she could not find a publisher, and had therefore decided to produce it herself. The current international symposium with several thousand delegates, provided an opportunity for her to publicise it, although she admitted that she had not had much of a response from the participants, who were nearly all men. The leaflet was basically a summary of a paper she was giving in one of the smaller conference rooms later in the day. She told me she lived in Sierra-Leone but that she and her husband also had a flat in London. I took her address. I suggested that she might submit the paper for publication in the British Journal of Family Planning.

She seemed mildly interested in the idea but not particularly enthusiastic. After my return to Glasgow I sent the leaflet to the Editor for her opinion. Her response was that the topic was of great interest but that the article would have to be properly prepared and presented for publication in a scientific journal. She wrote to this effect to Dr Koso-Thomas who eventually replied that she would see what she could do, but no article by her on female circumcision has ever been published in the British Journal of Family Planning, as far as I am aware.

Before I had left Britain, I arranged to meet a distinguished social anthropologist through a mutual friend. She had lived for several years with the Mende, an indigenous tribe in the Sierra-Leone hinterland and knew something of their customs and social structure. She explained that life for women is dominated by the Bundu, secret societies which are run by headwomen who are frequently the local Traditional Birth Attendants. Girls are initiated into the societies by circumcision performed by these forcible women. The Bundu are powerful throughout Sierra-Leone and their influence is not confined to the rural areas. It is almost impossible for a woman to reach any position of authority, or even find outside employment, unless she is an initiate and the practice is so deeply entrenched that even where the influence of the societies is less obvious, as in the capital, Freetown, circumcision is the norm.

Most of this urban population is Krio, that is, descended from the original freed slaves and subsequent early black colonists who interbred to some extent with Europeans of many nations. These people formed the first British colony in Africa and by the middle of the last century were exposed to strong Christian influence in the form of schools and hospitals founded, maintained and staffed by missionary societies and by the colonial power. By the end of Victoria's reign there were Krio doctors and lawyers and the beginnings of a Krio civil service. Anglican, Methodist and eventually Catholic churches were built, in unmistakable Victorian gothic style, all over Freetown and their congregations today would shame most in the mother country. Over the course of many generations there was a lot of intermarriage with indigenous people from up-country, many of whom were Muslim. Today the population of the capital is probably about seventy percent Christian. Whereas all the Muslim Krios participate in the ritual of circumcision, only some of the Christians do so. The better educated are less likely to comply but even they are subjected to a great deal of pressure and even physical violence.

Naturally, I told my anthropological friend of my acquaintance with Doctor Koso-Thomas, expecting to be told how helpful this contact would be. I was disconcerted to be warned against taking up her invitation when I reached Freetown.

"She has antagonised the Bundu by her campaign against female circumcision. She is not a native Sierra-Leonian and outsiders are not popular at the moment. She's married to the Vice-Chancellor of the University and knows all the politicians and the people that matter in Freetown but she has stirred up a very powerful hornets' nest over this issue. It is said that the past president's wife was probably the head of the most important Bundu Society in the country – I've no idea if that is true, but it gives you some idea of how these societies are perceived and how pervasive is their influence.

"If you are seen to be a friend of hers it may well be that the word will be spread about that you are not to be trusted and the clinics you work in could be black-listed."

This seemed to me to be a little over the top, but it did give me food for thought. I remembered her words three months later when I was being entertained in Olayinka's beautiful house, high on the crest of the escarpment overlooking Lumley beach. Perhaps fortunately, the power of the Bundu, in my case, was not put to the test, as I only visited that gracious establishment on that one occasion. Dr Koso-Thomas and her highly intelligent and cultured husband were frequently out of the country and our paths barely touched again.

One Sunday afternoon in March Lauretta brought her year old baby girl to tea with me in the flat. I had managed to buy some biscuits from Choitrams and had several bottles of Sprite cooling in a bucket of water in the shower, as I could not chill the drinks in the fridge because of the absence of power. Now that the ship delivering Calor Gas had arrived, I would be able to make a pot of tea. We sat comfortably chatting about why, and how, she had decided to take up nursing and whether it would be possible to up-grade her SECHN qualification to that of a fully registered nurse and midwife. The main problem was that she had left school without the necessary subjects and grades to admit her to the more prestigious and demanding course. Her family could not afford to pay the fees and continue to support her if she had stayed on at school to acquire them. She was a bright girl and I had worked with her long enough to be confident that she had the ability to gain the higher qualification but it seemed very unlikely that she would ever be able to keep herself and her daughter while she studied, let alone find the money for the fees. I felt we had got to know one another well enough for me to ask her a more personal question.

"Lauretta, what do you think about female circumcision?"

"It's a terrible thing to do to girls, I think it should be banned," she spoke with great feeling and there was obviously some personal experience behind her vehemence. I wondered if it would be too intrusive to ask her, when she forestalled me.

"My father is a Christian and so am I and my sisters. We don't believe in it and my father had forbidden my mother to allow it to be done to us but her mother, who lives up-country near Bo, she said we must be done or we would not be proper women."

"But surely you can't be circumcised against your will?"

"Oh yes you can. My mother tricked us. When we got back from school one day she said we had been invited to a party at my aunty's and we were to change into our best clothes. My younger sister didn't want to go and went out, so she escaped. We thought she was silly to miss the party. We went to my aunt's house on the outskirts of Freetown and as soon as we got there, I knew something was wrong. There were a lot of women who surrounded us and hustled us along to another house that was on its own. I guessed what was going to happen and screamed and tried to escape, but it was no good. I struggled and sat down on the ground but they lifted me up and carried me into this hut. There were other girls there who looked frightened, but they did nothing to help me. Then I was lifted onto a table and my legs were forced apart. All the time I was struggling and then an enormous fat women sat on my chest. Doctor Wilson, she was the fattest woman I have ever seen, I thought I was going to suffocate and I bit her buttock hard but it didn't stop them and I felt this agonising pain between my legs and knew I had been circumcised. My sister was done too."

"How old were you?"

"I was sixteen and my sister was nearly eighteen."

"Had you got a boy friend then?"

"Yes, and so had my sister but we hadn't had sex. That was one reason why my grandmother had made my mother get us done quickly, because it has to be done while you are still a virgin."

Some weeks later there was a general discussion among some of the other nurses while we were waiting for a meeting to begin. I had a great respect for Keturah who was an excellent field worker and had a special gift for communicating with the largely illiterate women in the markets and villages round the capital. She was a superb 'motivator' for the use of family planning and her skills had been used effectively in several local radio programmes. She had very different views on female circumcision.

"It's much more hygienic. How can you possibly be really clean when you've got all those bits of skin to wash? Germs get caught in the creases and I think any woman, or man for that matter, is dirty if they are not circumcised. Besides it is part of our culture in Sierra-Leone, the people who want to abolish it are outsiders, part of Western ways we don't want to copy."

Keturah is an intelligent woman whom I like and it was fascinating to me to hear her defend this appalling practice using a Western type argument based on hygienic considerations and bolstering it with an appeal to patriotism and a fierce defence of local custom against an alien culture. She is a Muslim Krio and well educated by local standards. She represents the views of a large proportion of educated women in Sierra-Leone and the eighty two percent of the population who are illiterate would agree with her, although their reasons for continuing the custom would not be so explicit. In the discussion that followed no-one mentioned the Bundu whose very existence must not be admitted in front of a stranger. I listened without contributing to the discussion, content to be an observer and thinking myself privileged to be there at all.

I do not think there is any possibility of abolishing female circumcision in Sierra-Leone in the foreseeable future and I think it would be foolish for any outside agency to try. The desire for change must come from within. As it is so closely bound up with the powerful hierarchy of the Bundu this will take a long time. The great mass of the people in Sierra-Leone are so cut off from the rest of the world media that most have little idea of what goes on outside the frontiers of their country. The lack of electricity for all but the very wealthy who can afford generators, means that there is no television. The local radio stations broadcast popular music (Western pop) with World, African and local news bulletins and some good educational items including several slots on health-related issues but reception was poor outside the capital and depended almost entirely on battery operated sets. The only batteries available locally were Chinese and had a maximum life of four hours, as I knew from personal experience. There were no outside newspapers and the local news sheets were so poorly written, spelt and printed that their content was suspected of being of the same quality (but they were a great source of amusement and were full of the latest gossip and scandal).

As only one in five people can read, Government policies concerning immunisation and AIDS were publicised by hoardings and posters which were of the 'every picture tells a story' kind with a brief message in words. One of these picturing a child obviously crippled by polio said in Krio 'UDAT BORN ME WAE NOR MARKLATE ME?' ('marklate' was the word for immunisation). This restricted access to what goes on in the rest of the world was confined to the illiterate as there was not a family I met amongst the educated, who did not have a relative, frequently several, who was living abroad in the UK, USA, or Canada. Many had been overseas themselves. Sylvia met and married her Sierra-Leonian husband in New York State when they were both students there. All Sister Cline's four children were either in the US or Canada; Sister Meux's husband was a surgeon who had lived and worked in New Jersey for fourteen years. Dr Ford's English wife lived with their family and worked as a nurse in Sheffield. Dr George Bernard Fraser had a house in Aberdeen, Scotland and his children were educated over there. Mr Brown, my unhelpful Indian landlord, owned a house in London which was let at a considerable profit when it was not being used by a member of his family to live in, while they studied some form of higher education.

Such professional families were largely Westernised and I am sure would not have wanted to have their daughters circumcised. But amongst the ruling political classes the attitudes would be different. Since independence and 'one man one vote' throughout the country, they were no longer predominantly Krio, but had tribal backgrounds in the Temne,

Mende, Limba and so on, and with many, the animist culture of their grandparents would be a strong influence. The Muslims could rightly point to the widespread practice of female circumcision in many Islamic countries, even although it is not part of the teaching of the Koran. There is nothing to motivate the Government to change its laissez-faire attitude and a great deal to maintaining the status quo.

Contrary to common perception in the West, the root of the problem lies with the women. Men have little to do with the perpetuation of the custom. I have yet to see a study of the relative rates of unfaithfulness between women with, and without, a clitoris. There appeared to be much the same changing of partners among the young women of Freetown as there was among the teenagers of Glasgow and I have no doubt the situation was similar among the married. Clitoridectomy has little to do with preventing sexual activity with more than one partner.

The most common form of mutilation I observed was absence of the clitoris which was the form of circumcision most widely practised among the Muslim Krios in Freetown. The other more extensive procedure involved removal of the labia minora as well. This was by no means uncommon, especially among women who had been born and brought up in the rural areas and who had come to the capital through marriage. Like the Irish born men resident in Glasgow, who used to go back to Galway and Donegal and, as the Pakistanis and Indians return now to the sub-continent, to find a wife, the Temne and Mende want to marry a woman from their own tribe up-country.

I only saw one woman who had suffered the most mutilating procedure of all, that is infibulation, in which not only the clitoris and labia minora are cut away but most of the labia majora are also removed and what remains of the two sides is stitched together leaving a small hole just large enough to allow urine and menstrual blood to escape. The young woman was a Limba, like her elderly husband, and came from the North, near the Guinea border. She was seventeen but had been married to her fifty year old husband for four years. She was his third wife and much younger than his other two wives but was in danger of being sent back to her parents because she had not yet borne a child. The old man must have been fond of her, because he brought her to the clinic and was prepared to spend a little money on Western medicine to see if that could help.

I have no doubt we were a last resort and that many visits had been made to indigenous practitioners and considerable sums had been spent on herbal and other more noisome native remedies, but the problem was basically a physical one. On examining her I found that she had been infibulated and that it was only possible to insert the tip of my index finger into the opening. It is true that it is possible for spermatozoa to swim from the vaginal opening to the cervix, and on, into the uterus and tube to fertilise an egg.

More than thirty years ago I had seen two women in Sheffield who were certainly pregnant and who were technically still virgins. They had paid a very unwelcome price for enjoying what used to be known as 'heavy petting', but it is very uncommon.

Four years of trying on her husband's part had not resulted in a pregnancy for this unfortunate young Limba girl. I explained the problem to them both, speaking English which Marjory, the nurse at Ports clinic that day, translated into Krio. The old man could understand it even though he was not a fluent speaker. He in turn spoke in Limba to his wife, at least, that is what Marjory thought it was. Fortunately the problem was one which could be explained fairly easily by using a spontaneously invented form of sign language. The hole was too small to allow penetration and had to be stretched to make it bigger. It was very important to do this gently and gradually over several weeks as, if it caused bleeding, it might close up again, tighter than ever.

"I will give you some special ointment to put on your finger to help you do this." I had been in West Africa long enough to know that it was the husband who had to be addressed and that he would be the one to perform the treatment.

"Put the end of your finger covered in the special ointment into the opening twice a day, except when your wife has her period. Then start to move your finger in the hole." I rotated my index finger inside the circle formed by approximating the tip of my finger and thumb of the other hand. "Then move it further inside until you can get it in beyond the second joint. Come back to see me in one month, four weeks today." We dispensed a tube of KY jelly, an inert but effective lubricant used by gynaecologists in more affluent societies to lubricate their gloved fingers before performing an internal examination. We used water, and sometimes a little soap, in our clinics, but I thought it was important to include a certain magic element which would enhance their belief in the efficacy of the treatment.

When they had gone I said to Marjory, "Do you think they will come back?"

"I don't know Doc, we'll have to wait and see," by which she indicated that she thought it was unlikely.

167

Four weeks later they returned looking pleased. The girl was all giggly smiles and it was hardly necessary for me to examine her to confirm that full intercourse had now taken place. No doubt it had been a very painful experience but she obviously thought it was well worth it. This story has a happy ending. On my last visit to Ports at the end of May the couple came back. She was about seven weeks pregnant and her smile was so infectious that we all, patients and staff alike, rejoiced with her. I felt I had to introduce a word of warning into the euphoria.

"When her time comes she must be delivered in the PCMH (Princess Christian Maternity Hospital). The tightness of the hole may hold back the head of the baby. If the birth is too long he may die and his mother may die also, so you must make sure she goes to hospital for the birth." I feared they were unlikely to follow this advice but hoped that the success of our treatment for their infertility might encourage him to bring her to our ante-natal clinic and we might even be able to refer her officially to the maternity hospital towards the end of her pregnancy.

Chapter 9 – April
How Am I Supposed to do My Work?

I RETURNED TO FREETOWN IN THE middle of April, after four weeks leave, to find that the country had been invaded by rebel Liberian soldiers belonging to Charles Taylor's faction. Sierra-Leone had been peripherally involved in the Liberian civil war before my arrival at the beginning of the previous August. The common boundary was a long one and impossible to defend, even if there had been the means and the will. Thousands of refugees had trickled over the border along the few, narrow, nearly impassable, roads and through the numerous tracks in the bush.

The very wealthy Liberians had flown out when it was still possible, to the USA or, if that was too difficult in the first rush of panic, to neighbouring African states like Guinea, Nigeria and the C'ote D'Ivoire. Many of the comfortably off had been driven over the frontier and along the three hundred miles of bush tracks and so called main roads to Freetown in their Mercedes and Peugeots, to take up residence in the three hotels on the Aberdeen peninsula. Most of them had moved on and now, in April, it was the presence of alien troops as well as the much greater prominence of the Sierra-Leonian army which I noticed.

In past months the going and coming of the troops of the West African Peace-Keeping Force by sea from the port, had become part of everyday life in the capital. On several occasions I had seen soldiers returning from a tour of duty in Liberia, instantly recognisable by their round white helmets, staggering up from the quayside laden with loot, a boy behind each carrying a television set and video-recorder and, on one occasion, a chest freezer on a cart.

Now the troops were everywhere, and were stationed in and around the capital. Rumours were rife. Every day one member of staff or another came in to work with hair-raising stories of imminent disaster – the Aberdeen peninsula was going to be invaded; an advance party of rebels had been seen in Wellington; an uncle had been up a palm tree tapping for palm wine and had seen a group of armed men bury their weapons under a bush on the outskirts of Freetown.

In spite of these alarms, work went on as usual and each week we travelled the fifteen miles to Hastings, Grafton and Jui. Beside the turn-off to Grafton a large body of Nigerian troops was encamped. It seemed to take several weeks to become fully established, but the local grapevine informed us that this was the base-camp for the counter measures to be taken against the invading rebels.

More personally alarming were the spot checks and road blocks set up by the army in residential areas at night. It was somewhat disconcerting to be ordered out of one's car when returning home from a visit to friends and asked to open the boot so that it could be searched. The G.O.C. of the Sierra-Leonian army lived in this area, and I expect the troops had orders to stop every vehicle entering or leaving it. But the possibility that Leona or myself would be smuggling an armed rebel or his weapons into the heart of the wealthier suburbs, was patently absurd. There was no doubt that the men enjoyed asking two elderly Western ladies to get out of their car (we were sharing our transport on the first occasion) at gun point but they were friendly, in a drunken sort of way, and we responded with good-humour and a joke about hiding bombs in the boot. It was their intoxicated state which alarmed us. They waved their weapons about with careless abandon and one felt that if we had said, or done, anything which upset even one of them, a trigger-happy finger would have sprayed out a stream of death without a second thought.

There were other changes within the Marie-Stopes organisation. Two Liberian trained women doctors were employed on a semi-permanent basis. I came to have a high opinion of them both and I was relieved to know there was no possibility of the Russian doctor returning to our ranks. The unsatisfactory situation at the Kissy clinic had been sorted out by not renewing the temporary contract of the senior nurse, who had been found to be charging patients and pocketing the fees without entering their attendances in the register. No wonder the numbers appeared to have fallen and the nurses were so disgruntled when I was there on Fridays. They would have told the clients not to come on that day of the week, no doubt spreading some unpleasant rumour of my incompetence or callousness. The SECHN was easily led. She had been moved to another clinic under the eagle eye of Sister Meux. Since then the number of patients had gone up steadily and the session was now more than covering its costs.

Grafton had not changed much in my absence. We were seeing more patients, probably because the Aid organisation that had distributed free medicines (but not contraception or ante-natal care) weekly, on Fridays, had stopped coming.

A tall thin woman, very pregnant, came in for the first time. She had no idea of the date of her last period, which was quite usual for the Africans living out of town. They would be able to tell you the timing of their last period if this was within the past three months by reference to the moon. They would often count on their fingers, lifting one finger up and raising their eyes heavenward every time they mentally ticked off a full moon. Once they were pregnant, although they could not name the month in which the child was due, they were almost invariably right about how long it would be before the child would be born.

"How many pikins you born?" she was asked.

"One, heah," she indicated the three year old boy holding onto her skirt.

"How old is he?"

"Three years, Sistah."

"Get up on that couch and I feel the belly." The woman climbed up with some difficulty and Sister palpated her abdomen. Fortunately they agreed that the baby was due sometime in the next week but, less fortunately, it was obvious that there was a major problem. The head was not down in the pelvis, nicely positioned for a vertex (ie head first) delivery but was lying across her body with the head in one flank and the feet easily felt in the other. This is known as a 'transverse lie' and unless successfully corrected it would be impossible for the child to be born through the vagina. Its survival, and probably that of its mother, would depend on a caesarian section. Even if Sister 'turned' the baby in utero now, it was virtually certain that it would rotate back to its present position well before delivery. In this case, the woman's muscles were so slack and the foetus was lying so high in her abdomen that we both thought there was probably some mass in the pelvis which was preventing it from assuming the normal position.

"You must go to the hospital to have the baby. It would be better if you went soon, before you are in labour so that they know about you before it is an emergency." Sister then explained to her exactly why this was so important and why she would almost certainly need an operation. The patient listened quietly and nodded her head at intervals.

"Yes, Sistah they tell me all last time," she said.

"What do you mean, 'last time'?" queried the nurse.

171

"Last time I was in Princess Christian (the maternity hospital)," she replied.

"But you said you only had one pikin, and here he is, fine boy, nothing went wrong when he was born did it?" Sister was getting a little annoyed at the discrepancies in the story.

"Sistah, you asked me how many pikins I got. I got one. The last baby, he born dead. They had to cut him to get him out of me but he was dead before that. His arm came out first and it wouldn't go back and he was stuck fast. I know about what you tell me."

All we could do was to emphasise that she MUST go to the hospital as soon as she thought she was in labour even if this meant going in a taxi the twenty miles to the city and that she might die if she did not have an operation. Her husband must find the money from somewhere.

The next patient was also attending for the first time for ante-natal care. This would be her eleventh confinement, as far as she could remember. She had six living children but her last baby had been born dead. She lay on the couch and Sister felt her abdomen.

"The head is beginning to engage, with such high parity I don't think she'll go much longer," she said. "I'll take her blood pressure now and then we'll send her with a note to get her blood checked and her urine tested." She wrapped the cuff of the sphygmomanometer round the woman's upper arm. Of all the Marie-Stopes staff she was the one whose expression was the most difficult to interpret. She usually kept her thoughts to herself but when she did smile it was worth waiting for. On this occasion her dead-pan look was broken by a minimal downward twitch of her lips.

"Would you mind checking this for me, Doctor?" she asked.

I repeated the procedure with what proved to be the same result. The patient's blood pressure was 210 over 160. The upper limits of normal, especially in pregnant women are 120 over 90. This lady had very severe hypertension which could easily cause her death before or during labour, and would probably result in the baby dying too. High blood pressure occurring late in pregnancy is known as pre-eclamptic toxaemia and is more common with first babies. This patient had had many successful deliveries, although the last had ended in disaster. It seemed to me more likely that she had developed her hypertension independently of the pregnancy and had probably suffered from it for several years, as it is a very common problem amongst West Africans of both sexes. Whatever the causes, her present condition was very serious and she needed immediate induction or preferably a caesarean section. We tried to explain this to her but it was difficult because, apart from admitting to a headache, she said she was not ill and therefore saw no need to go to the hospital that day.

"Besides," she said in Krio, "My man is not back from his work until 6 o'clock and I have no money." This is an unanswerable argument as no money = no operation, and I had seen a woman die in the maternity hospital from obstructed labour because her relatives did not arrive in time with the cash. All we could do was emphasise that if she wanted this child to have a chance of life, and of surviving herself, she must go to the Princess Christian Maternity Hospital as soon as possible and take enough money to pay for an operation, even if they had to borrow it.

It was now after half past four and we still had to collect Keturah from Jui before we started the long drive back, but another patient had arrived while we were attending to the last one. She was grossly obese and had great difficulty in walking. She looked a thoroughly disagreeable old woman and my heart sank as she lowered herself with considerable difficulty onto the inadequate chair.

"What de problem Mammie?" I asked her.

"My leg, it's my leg." Both enormous extremities were extended in front of her like two huge tree trunks but when I pulled up her skirt I could see that one was even bigger than the other and, that in addition to the layers of fat encasing the limb, the skin was grossly distended with fluid. Her entire leg looked like one of those sausage-dog balloons that are blown up and twisted to separate the body from the head, as the skin was tightly creased at her knee and ankle. It was also reddened and very painful down the back of her calf. I had no doubt she had a thrombosis, a clot, in the main vein at the back of her leg. She yelled so loudly when I touched her that I made no attempt to see if I could feel the thrombosed vein in her thigh. It would have been almost impossible through all those layers of adipose tissue, even if she had been co-operative. The important thing was to try and prevent the clot from extending further up, as it could eventually block the entire venous drainage from her leg. The immediate risk was from a bit of clot breaking off and being carried into the blood vessels going to the lungs, (a pulmonary embolism) as this can be fatal.

It was no good thinking about hospitalisation and intravenous anti-coagulants with the dose controlled by sophisticated blood tests. Aspirin was cheap and available and has proved effective in reducing attacks of coronary thrombosis by its ability to keep the blood fluid. I prescribed two aspirins straight away, to be followed by one night and morning until we returned the next week. She was given an immediate injection of penicillin for its psychological effect, as the old beldame would not have thought she had been properly treated unless she had a 'chook' and would therefore not have taken the aspirin which was what she needed. Two diuretic tablets were dispensed to take every other morning to help to reduce the swelling and the tension in the skin.

"And Mammie, most important, you go home and you rest, and you put your leg up and you don't walk except when you go to the toilet. You understand?"

"And how am I supposed to do my work if I cannot walk?"

"What work do you do?" I asked.

"I am the TBA," she announced. Sister and I looked at one another. TBA, 'traditional birth attendant'; in other words, she was the midwife! If our two previous patients failed to go to the hospital, they would be in the care of this monstrous and disabled old woman.

She grunted and grumbled to herself, but she was in too much pain not to know that what the doctor said was also common sense.

It was after 5.00 before we finally drove away and nearly 7.00 before we arrived in Adelaide Street. It had taken forty minutes to drive along the mile of Kissy Road because, as usually happened if we arrived there after 4.30, we had met a Muslim funeral processing literally at funereal pace on its way to the huge municipal cemetery. This one had been even longer than normal and the men and boys straggled slowly along surrounding and behind the coffin, occupying more than half the width of the street. It was dark by the time I reached home, but how I enjoyed my shower, even if it was by the light of a single candle.

I looked forward with professional interest to the following Tuesday. Both our ladies had delivered, the first had gone to hospital the next day and had had a caesarian section, she and her baby were well; the hypertensive patient had gone into labour that evening and had delivered herself at home without any problems. So much for our gloomy forebodings. Her blood pressure remained sky-high and she had been very lucky to have got away with it. Even the TBA was much improved and agreed to continue taking half an aspirin a day for the next three months. Whether she would or not, I could not assess but at least she gave us a grudging smile.

One Thursday evening at the golf club a pleasant English woman came up to me. Her husband managed one of the few remaining businesses in

Freetown and I knew she lived in one of the modern company houses on the Loop near the British High Commission compound.

"My steward's little boy hasn't been well for months, I wondered if I could send him down to your clinic?"

"Of course, no problem. We have sessions every day at Collegiate School Road," I replied.

"Yes, but I would really like you to see him yourself. His father has already taken him to a private doctor but, apart from a huge bill for antibiotics and vitamins, there has been nothing to show for it and the child is no better."

I was quite prepared to arrange to see the little boy at one of my usual sessions but I added, "I am not a paediatrician, and I'll probably do no better than the previous doctor, but it won't cost you anything like so much."

The following week the child arrived with his father in the company Peugeot. All the staff and the few remaining patients, were agog at the arrival of this private limousine. I had deliberately suggested a time in the early afternoon when we were least likely to be busy and waiting time would be minimal. He was four years old and very underweight for his age. I knew his diet was not the problem, but his father said his appetite was very poor. He also had an irritating cough especially at night.

"Has he had all his marklate?" I asked. 'Marklate' is the Krio term for immunisation. UNICEF, with funding from Italy and the official collaboration of the Sierra-Leone Ministry of Health had put an enormous effort into a mass immunisation campaign which had been remarkably successful. It was claimed that over seventy percent of the pre-school children in Freetown were fully immunised, including BCG at birth to protect them against tuberculosis. Usman's father was quite indignant that I should even ask.

"Of course, Doctor, he has had all his chooks. He was a fine boy until six months ago and now he is wasting away. He has no spirit, he doesn't want to play anymore."

I listened to the little boy's chest and was far from happy with what I heard. I wrote a note to the radiologist at his rooms in Bathurst Street. "Usman Koromah, 4 years. Chronic cough, failure to thrive? Koch's infection. Chest X-ray please." I had deliberately used the medical euphemism 'Koch's infection' instead of 'tuberculosis' because, if I was wrong, I did not want the child's parents to suffer the unnecessary anxiety of thinking that that was what was wrong. Mr Koromah was an intelligent literate man and would understand the implications of a diagnosis of

TB. If I was right, I wanted to tell his parents myself, if possible, and be able to emphasise the positive side. As his employer was paying the costs of the child's medical care, I knew the test would be done without delay. I was by now aware that vaccination with BCG did not always confer immunity. I had seen two other children in the past month who had active pulmonary tuberculosis in spite of being immunised against it.

The other spectre in the back of my mind was AIDS. In many other parts of Africa the resurgence of TB was a direct consequence of the victim's depressed immunity associated with HIV infection. I had not seen any patients, so far, that I thought were suffering from AIDS but the possibility was always in my mind. In Usman's case the obvious thing to do was to ask about the health of his mother, whom I had not seen.

"How is the boy's mother?" I asked. "Is she quite healthy?" I had wondered whether it was because his mother was sick, that she had not accompanied the child.

"She is very fine Doctor, but it is right for a father to be with his son and discuss the problem with the doctor. Usman is my only child and his health is very important to me." This almost certainly ruled out AIDS and I would have expected him to have become ill before this if he was suffering from a congenital infection handed on from his mother.

When they arrived at the clinic Mr Koromah was holding a large brown envelope containing Usman's chest X-ray. The report was scribbled on the back of my referral note.

"Bilateral pulmonary tuberculosis." I do not know whether his father had read it and did not ask.

"Usman has got TB in his lungs but nowadays this can be cured. It will take several months, but by next Christmas he will be well again and long before that he will be running about and eating properly like his old self."

To my surprise his father smiled. "It is good to know the name of his illness especially as you say he will get better. I was afraid it was something no medicine could cure when the other doctor said it was just a cold on his chest, but his treatment did no good."

"I'm afraid he will have to have chooks every day for at least eight weeks and he won't like that. He's also got to take tablets for probably six months but, if you make sure he gets the treatment regularly, he will get well. Otherwise he will die." I spoke sternly as I wanted the man to realise that consistent treatment was essential. Fortunately there were two important factors in the present situation which made the prognosis good. Firstly my friend, his employer, would pay for all the drugs, clinic attendances and X-rays that would be needed. Sadly, lack of money to cover the necessary treatment over the mandatory six months meant that there were a lot of defaulters who not only relapsed themselves, but increased the likelihood of producing strains of the bacillus that were resistant to routine drugs. Secondly, she would encourage the parents to persevere in keeping up the treatment, especially when he began to improve and put on weight and they would naturally think he was cured and did not need any more drugs.

When I left Sierra-Leone two months later Usman was a normal energetic cheerful five year old, he had gained weight and was measurably taller, but he still had four months of tablet taking ahead of him to make sure the disease was completely eliminated.

Not long after my return I had a stupid accident. I tripped in my flat and fell against the wall on the point of my left shoulder. As I hit it, I heard the muscle fibres rip with a noise like tearing canvas. Although it was painful I was not shocked and was able to reach the wash-basin to give my grazed knees a good clean with soap and water. I did not want tropical ulcers developing from infected lesions and, in practice, they healed very quickly. My shoulder was another matter. I was certain that I had neither dislocated the joint nor broken any bones but it was very painful and I could not raise my arm above waist level. I thought, correctly, that I had torn the deltoid and triceps muscles which are used to move the arms away from the sides and above the head. I also thought, mistakenly, that the injury would recover in a week or ten days. Fortunately the mishap occurred on a Friday and I was over the worst discomfort by Monday, but found it was impossible to drive. I had tried sitting in the car on Sunday afternoon and could only just manage to rest my left hand on the lowest part of the steering wheel. In Sierra-Leone one drives on the right and the Fiesta was a right-hand drive car so that I would need to control the steering with my left hand while using my right to change gear and use the handbrake. It was no good. I used Mrs Brown's telephone to speak to Sylvia in the office and asked her if she could arrange for me to be picked up by the Land-Rover to be taken to work.

This was the beginning of a tedious time. It was two months before I could drive again and by that time I was back in Scotland. There was one great improvement in my living conditions which almost compensated for having to be dependent on a driver for my transport. Sylvia had bought a small petrol generator which was connected to my electricity circuit. When filled with two-thirds of a gallon of fuel it would

177

run for three hours. I soon became an expert at estimating how much petrol would be needed for a given length of time. If I was going out for the evening I would half fill it, have it on from 6.45 to 7.30 and restart it when I returned so that I would not have to go to bed in the dark.

More often than not, I was home. I filled the generator, usually by torchlight as it was dark by 7 o'clock in James' old sleeping quarters between the concrete walls. I used a funnel, which was not easy when my left arm was useless above waist level, and a five gallon drum is quite a weight. Then the starting rope had to be firmly jerked to activate the motor. I had to do this with my right arm and as I am left-handed, I was always afraid that I would not have the power to get it going. Every night I had a fleeting moment of despair before the engine coughed and sometimes stumbled before the roar which preceded its noisy rhythmical chug, like the heart beat of heaven to me on some of those long evenings. I knew the fuel would run out in three hours and I planned my activities carefully – reading or writing letters or preparing talks for the training courses we were running in the normality of electric light and the coolness of the air-conditioner.

At 9.30 it was time to prepare for bed. I enjoyed a cold shower, put on my nightie and slipped my feet into a pair of sandals, not because the floor was dirty, but the cockroaches were ubiquitous and I had a horror of scrunching one with my bare foot. I checked that everything I would need when the light went out was in its place on the small bookshelf along the side of my bed. I inserted the tape I wanted to hear in the cassette player and placed the torch beside it. Then it was time to tuck myself inside the cocoon of mattress and enfolding mosquito net, remembering to take my book inside with me. Many a night I would curse with frustration when I had at last got myself comfortably and effectively tucked up, only to realise that I had left my current volume of light literature on the table on the other side of the room. When all was well, I probably had five or ten minutes to read before the fuel ran out at 10 o'clock and the room would black out without warning. The book would be pushed under the pillow and I would carefully extend my hand between mattress and net and switch on the cassette. One side of one tape was usually long enough to listen to, without falling asleep and forgetting to turn off the machine, which would have been a waste of my precious batteries.

Chapter 10 – May
I Think He's Dead. . .

My time in Sierra-Leone was nearly over. My shoulder was taking longer to mend than I had anticipated. Although I subsequently discovered my initial optimism had been ill-founded I did not want to consult a local specialist, in case some surgical intervention was suggested which I would not have contemplated in Freetown. In any case I was sure that time and active physiotherapy were what was required. In practice, the latter was only available in the UK.

The two Liberian doctors were good and well established in the Marie-Stopes organisation so that my departure a few weeks earlier than had been originally intended, would not damage clinic services. We were involved in two training programmes, one for our own staff, who, we hoped, would be able to restart the clinic at Segwemba when the trouble with the invading rebels had subsided (this never happened as the district remained too dangerous to allow staff to work there). The second was for the doctor and nursing staff of the Aid agency that had approached us in January. It was starting a primary health care project up-country and wanted to include family planning in its programme. I was anxious to complete these courses before I left and booked my flight back for the end of May.

I continued to attend clinic sessions whenever there was a gap in the training programme but the highlights of my last fortnight were two separate events to mark my impending departure. I was tempted to write 'celebrate', but this would give an entirely erroneous impression. They were happy occasions for a sad reason. The first was the Farewell Ceremony held at the Milton Margai School for the Blind.

The entire school was assembled in one of the classrooms, wearing their best freshly laundered uniform dresses, shirts and shorts in bright yellow cotton. The Headmaster opened the ceremony in his rich, mellifluous voice.

179

"Today is Tuesday the 28 May 1991, and we are gathered here today to say farewell to a very good friend of ours, Doctor Libby Wilson. . . " He thanked me in embarrassingly laudatory terms for the medical care I had given the children of the school. He remembered that I had managed to treat the 'wounds' on their legs so that they were all healed in time for the annual prize-giving and he spoke of Fatu, who had died in spite of all our efforts. . .

I was entertained by singing and music – rhythmic clapping is an essential part of any African music – and then a superbly performed play. This included a graphic portrayal of what is probably Soloman's most well-publicised judgement concerning the female parentage of a baby.

" . . . the baby is mine, last night when I was busy looking after my baby she went out leaving her baby all alone. She came home quite drunk, not caring about her child. In the morning when she discovered that her baby was dead, she accused me of stealing her baby. . ." There was more than a touch of realism about this part of the scenario. The young presenters played their parts with gusto and spoke clearly and with a total lack of self-consciousness which was very enjoyable.

When the play was over the whole school sang the school song whose words and music had been composed by the Headmaster.

We are the pupils of the Milton Margai School
For the blind in Sierra-Leone
We cannot see but we will conquer
So that we may take our place, as people of the race.

The tune was stirring, the part-singing musically satisfying and their enthusiasm moved me greatly. To see and hear these blind children singing so confidently of taking their place in the world outside, when I knew the reality for most of them would be hardship and deprivation, made it difficult for me to maintain my composure.

It was my turn next. I am afraid my words lacked the oratory of the Headmaster but the sentiments were genuine. I HAD looked forward to my visits to the school, " . . . not because I wanted you to be sick but because I enjoyed meeting you and saying 'Hello'."

After I had been personally thanked by the head-boy, and each of the staff had expressed their best wishes for my journey home and future happiness, the ceremony ended in a prayer in which I was asked through the Heavenly Intermediary not to forget the Milton Margai School for the blind in Freetown, Sallone. He must have responded to their supplication as I remember them vividly and with great affection and keep in touch through VSO.

The second 'celebration' was the party given by Sylvia and the Marie-Stopes staff to bid me farewell, but before this had taken place there was a more disturbing episode.

Ten days before I was due to return home, I was reading in my room when there was a loud knock on the door. I opened up to find Leona on the threshold.

"Libby, can you come with me at once? It's Robert, I think he's dead." Without delay I padlocked the door behind me and followed her up the side of the house onto the main road, where she had parked her CRS Peugeot outside the Kingdom Hall.

"A boy brought a message to me from Mrs Johnson to say Robert would not wake up and would I go at once?"

I remembered that Mrs Johnson was the sensible retired school-mistress who lived in Aberdeen who had been a good friend of Robert's mother when she spent nearly four months living with her son in the village. Muriel had become increasingly weak and ill and eventually I had had to insist that she return to Devon before she became too feeble to walk across to the aircraft and mount the steps to the cabin. She soon regained her strength and, somewhat to her dismay, the two and a half stone she had lost in her fifteen weeks in Freetown, once she returned to her comfortable little home in the west country.

Leona explained that she had taken the boy back with her in the car while he told her all that he knew. Robert had been dropped off by the CRS vehicle about 4.45 at the end of his day's work. At 5.30 the boy had called in to his house to see if he wanted any jobs doing, or if he wanted a cup of tea. Robert was lying on his bed, apparently asleep, but the boy could not rouse him. Like most of the population of Aberdeen in an emergency, he ran across to seek the help of Mrs Johnson who went back to the house with him. She knew Robert was employed by the Catholic Aid Society and that his boss was Sister Leona who lived in the Bintumani. The boy was sent to the hotel to fetch her.

All these too-ings and fro-ings had taken some time and it was well after 7.00 before Leona had her first sight of what she was certain was a dead man. She left the boy to keep guard while she came for me, knowing that a doctor would be needed to certify death, even if it was too late to save his life.

We turned off the tarmaced road onto the dirt track that led into the village, slithering and skidding on the loose rubble that had been tipped into the worse craters in the steep surface. Leona parked outside the house and we stepped up onto the veranda, where the boy was standing quietly in the shadows. We opened the front door and stepped carefully over the plastic water pipes lying carelessly on the uneven concrete, walked round the mound of sand in the corner of the room which had been sitting there since my first visit to the house six months before, waiting for Robert to skim the floor when he had saved enough money to finish the job, and went through the doorless opening into the bedroom.

Leona had a torch by means of which we were able to find our way round the obstacles, but it was a poor substitute for electric light when it came to examining the situation in front of us. The shallow bed-frame bearing the double mattress sat directly on the concrete floor, on which lay the body of a middle-aged man. He was dressed and lying peacefully on his back with his eyes open, his left arm slightly bent across his lower trunk, the right half hanging over the side of the bed, his hand a few inches above a mug which lay tipped over on the floor. He looked very peaceful, his face unlined in the torch light and no signs of pain or distress in the position of his limbs, no rucking of the sheet or displacement of the pillow.

There was no doubt that he was dead. Indeed the body was already beginning to cool. I looked carefully at his conjunctiva and round and inside his mouth to make sure there were no petechial haemorrhages which might indicate smothering and round his neck to eliminate the possibility of strangulation by ligature. I undid his shirt and the top of his trousers but could find no sign of a wound.

"Would you mind helping me to turn him onto his side?" I asked Leona. Together we gently rolled the body over so that I could examine the back as carefully as I had looked at the front. I could find nothing to suggest foul play. We laid him once more to rest on his back. I picked up the mug. There was still a small puddle of what looked like tea drying up on the floor. It contained no residue of powdered tablets or remains of capsules.

"We have to be sure there are no signs of third party interference," I said. "We know there have been some unpleasant goings-on here in the past and we've got to be certain there was no hanky-panky about this death."

"What next?" asked Leona.

"Well, he was a British citizen and I think the British High Commission must take over responsibility now," I replied.

"Then," she said, "I'd better get Rick (her second-in-command) to come and look after things here."

We closed the door and told the patient waiter on the veranda that his vigil would soon be over, as we were going to fetch some-one to take over from him. We bumped our way down onto the main road and Leona managed to find Rick's apartment in Murray Town without too much delay. He had already gone to bed, but once roused, grasped the situation quickly and went off to Aberdeen to hold the fort. We went up the hill to the British High Commission compound to seek out David Emery. Fortunately he was at home and, while we explained the reason for our untimely visit, his wife made us welcome and gave us cold drinks.

David at first seemed reluctant to become involved and appeared to be throwing out hints that perhaps Robert's American employers might be the people to make the necessary arrangements. I was beginning to feel a little uncomfortable and broke in.

"But surely this is the responsibility of the High Commission? Robert was a British citizen and if a British citizen dies abroad and has no relatives in the country it is OUR duty to look after his interests. We can't expect other people to do it for us. Wasn't an English VSO drowned up-country last year? I remember being told about how difficult it was to make the arrangements when that happened. At least Robert has died in Freetown."

"Yes, of course it's our responsibility," David replied. "I only meant that Leona knows a lot more about his family situation and we would be very grateful for all the help she can give us. Now, have you informed the police?"

We drove back down the hill and along the beach road to the Aberdeen police station which showed no signs of closing down for the night. David, Leona and I went into the open reception area and spoke to a tall sergeant on duty. He greeted me with, "Hello Doctor, what's the problem?" which was a nice inversion of our previous roles. I explained our difficulty.

"OK, wait," he said. "I phone Headquarters." He got through remarkably quickly, spoke and listened for a moment or two. "No funny games?" he asked.

"No signs of funny games or foul play," I said firmly. He relayed this message to his superior, listened again and put the phone down.

"It's OK, there is no need for a post-mortem. You can take the body."

This of course was exactly what we could not do. No arrangements for its disposal could be made without consulting Robert's mother who was his next of kin and was living in Devonshire. It would probably take four days to receive a reply from her and in the meantime bodies do not keep well in the tropics when there are no facilities for refrigeration.

The police were able to give David the name and address of an all-night undertaker and he went off to contact them.

"Wait for me here," he suggested, as it would be necessary for us to guide the undertaker's van to the house where the body lay.

Leona and I sat in the car with the windows down in the bright moonlight, outside the police station. A lanky young policeman in uniform draped himself against the windscreen,

"Doctor, me body dey ache, I have big big urrm (worm) in de belleh."

"Right Abu, you come see me Wednesday, I give you medicine then. I got no medicine now." As this was obviously true, he wandered off and a short time later I had a more rewarding conversation. This young man's wife had consulted me at the Aberdeen clinic a week or two before with a nasty infection in her arm. It required a special type of antibiotic which was expensive and not normally available in our clinics but I had brought a supply out with me from home for my personal use, if I should require it. As I was going home in the near future and had not needed it, I was glad to be able to give it to her. Happily it had worked quickly and effectively and his wife was now quite well. I had met him before when I had handed the drug in to the police station for him to collect on the evening of the day I had seen her. It was necessary to get the treatment started as soon as possible and the simplest plan was for me to deliver it when I was on my way to meet Leona for our evening out together. The young policeman had been amazed that I had gone to so much trouble, little enough in practice but he wanted to thank me.

"I think you'd better start a midnight clinic here, Libby," remarked Leona laughing in spite of the sombre reason for our presence outside a police station at such an unsociable hour.

Eventually the lights of the BHC Land-Rover, followed by a type of estate-car, were seen approaching. I knew that the crunch was about to come. We all got out of our vehicles and the undertaker confirmed that the only way of preserving the body long enough for Robert's mother to let her wishes be known, was to have it embalmed. David made it clear that there was no way in which he could authorise the payment by the BHC of the modest sum required (something like £50). I found out later that the local form of embalming was not the Tut-en-Khamun procedure, with viscera enclosed in canopic jars and the body bound in bandages, but the injection of sufficient formaldehyde to prevent the immediate decomposition of the corpse. But the undertaker required to deal with the matter immediately and had to be paid.

"For lands sakes," said Leona, "CRS will pay for it. It's only a hundred dollars and he was an employee, even if not on the permanent staff. We can't all stand here arguing among ourselves while the poor fellow's body is still lying on his bed."

As this settled the matter, we re-embarked and set off in convoy to the house in Aberdeen village. There was a large silent crowd of Africans outside the building. Robert had been well liked and, in the uncanny way that news travels round a small community, most of the neighbourhood had gathered to watch his last journey from home. They were respectful and dignified. Mrs Johnson came over and spoke to us quietly. She was obviously distressed.

"His poor Mother, she is such a sweet lady and Robert was her only son."

Leona and I waited outside while the undertaker's men went in and did what was needed. It did not take long and they soon came out bearing a long burden enclosed in plastic sheeting which was placed decently in the 'hearse' and driven off. Leona drove me home and I finally crawled under my mosquito net at a quarter to one, but this was only the end of the beginning for those of us involved in Robert's obsequies.

The next day I went up to the Emery's house at tea-time to sign the death certificate.

"What was the cause of death?" David asked, not for the first time. This was the question that had been in the forefront of my mind since my first sight of Robert's obviously dead body in the torch-light the night before. The possibility of foul play was a real one. I knew that he had had a confrontation a few weeks before with a rather unsavoury character who, at one time, appeared to have some hold over him. This man had had free access to the house and had been caught stealing building materials from the premises. His younger brother had remained on good terms with Robert and had been very helpful when Mrs Morton was convalescent prior to her departure for England. In addition, Robert always seemed to be short of money and was known to be in debt. His landlord had lived in the upper and airier half of the house. He was a retired police officer but had recently been found to be diabetic. He had been a good neighbour and Robert had been distressed when the man died in what was thought to be a diabetic coma at a weekend three or four weeks before. In spite of all his family and Robert could do, no doctor could be found who would come out and visit him. There had been a post-mortem and it was understood that death had been due to natural causes but a faint whiff of suspicion had remained, especially as it had been Mr Tarawalli's goods that had been stolen.

Once I had eliminated murder, the possibility of suicide by overdosage with a drug remained. I felt that psychologically this was quite possible as Robert had had a lot on his mind, especially with regard to his cash flow problems and, although he was far from introverted at work, he had no close friends.

I did not go into details of my original fears about foul play but I needed to explain why I thought suicide was ruled out in spite of general considerations regarding his state of mind.

"I do not know of any drug that can be taken by mouth, which acts by sending one to sleep, and which would kill in an hour and a half."

"What about injecting himself?" asked David.

"No syringe, no needle, no ampoules, no sign of any kind of tourniquet. No, I'm sure that is not a realistic suggestion."

Robert had been unconscious by 5.30. It appeared that he had come in from work, made himself a cup of tea on the paraffin stove and had lain down on his bed, the mug slipping out of his flaccid grasp as he had become rapidly comatose. There was no bottle of tablets or capsules, no sediment in the mug or in the puddle on the floor and no trace of powder or half swallowed medicaments in or round his mouth.

"Then why did he die?" David, not unreasonably, reiterated.

"I think he must have had a cerebral haemorrhage. Leona told me today that his colleagues at CRS said he was complaining of a bad headache when he was dropped off – of course he did suffer from migraine and so this was nothing out of the usual for him, but it was probably the onset of the bleeding inside his head."

"I thought he was too young to have something like that. After all he was only about fifty."

"Some people have tiny weak places in the walls of the blood vessels round the base of the brain. The pressure inside the artery gradually expands the weakened outer wall so that it forms a little balloon. They're usually quite small and round and so they are called 'berry' aneurysms."

"Surely, if you know they are there you can have treatment for them?" said David.

"The trouble is that most people have no idea they have anything wrong. They feel quite well, although, of course, if the balloons get big they may press on other structures nearby and cause symptoms and recurrent headaches could be a warning. If the aneurysm bursts it can be catastrophic and cause death, although many nowadays are diagnosed in time and operated on. Of course, here in Sierra-Leone, even if he had been found before his death, nobody could have done anything to save him, there just aren't the facilities. Even at home in England he obviously died so quickly that he wouldn't have got to the necessary specialised neuro-surgical unit in time.

"So what are you going to put on the death certificate?" asked David.

"Cerebral haemorrhage," I replied without hesitation. "That is the only reasonable diagnosis."

"We certainly don't want to raise any questions in anyone else's mind," said the diplomat.

"My main concern is with the living, and that means Mrs Morton. It is important that she knows her son died from natural causes and that no-one is to blame, especially not Robert himself. I know you've been making arrangements to contact her – what do you actually do in cases like this?"

"We've contacted the Home Office by fax, some-one in Leona's office had Robert's sister's address so the police are going to contact her and arrange for her to break the news to his mother. I understand she has a heart condition and isn't very strong? Once we get a message from her, we will know whether to ship the body home or bury it here." Neither prospect seemed very inviting to David.

"I'm sure she won't want him shipped or air-lifted home," I replied. "She's a sensible woman, not very well off and Robert hasn't lived at home properly for some time, so it's not as though he has lots of friends waiting to pay their last respects. I'm very glad she managed to come out here and stay with him (even if it did nearly kill her, I added to myself). She's only been home two months and I think the memories she has will be more important to her than burying his body in Devonshire."

I signed the death certificate and three days later a message came from Muriel that she wanted Robert buried in Sierra-Leone, a country he had felt almost more at home in than in England. Naturally, there had already been considerable discussion about what should be done if it was decided to bury him in Freetown. It was agreed that the Commonwealth War Grave Cemetery by the sea should be his last resting place, beside a few other civilians who had died working for the people of this impoverished land, and the servicemen who had been buried there as a result of war.

I was leaving for Scotland on the Thursday KLM flight but, unfortunately, the funeral had to be held on the Friday as many of his CRS colleagues were up-country and were not coming back until the day before. Leona told me that the police had changed their minds about the necessity for a post-mortem. I admit that this did make me somewhat apprehensive. I was as sure as I could be that Robert had died of a cerebral haemorrhage, but there was always the possibility that I had missed something. I resolutely tried to put the probable consequences of an incorrect death certificate out of my mind. Delayed departure was the most likely and the least unpleasant.

In the end, it was never put to the test. No-one would pay the pathologist to do the post-mortem. The British High Commission firmly refused and, knowing when the cause was lost, the police then put pressure on the Catholic Aid Society in the person of Leona. Perhaps they thought a middle-aged nun would be easier to persuade than a younger male diplomat. How wrong they were.

"Why should an American charity spend its funds on a post-mortem examination of an Englishman who was not even on our permanent staff? If the police want the examination, go right ahead and do it. It's nothing to do with us!"

The police wanted the post-mortem but not enough to pay for it, so Robert's body was not subjected to further indignities and the funeral arrangements went ahead without interruption. I did not feel entirely easy in my mind until I was safely in the aircraft en route for Amsterdam and home. Leona managed to give me a printed sheet of the service that was to be held the next day and, on my arrival at Heathrow, I posted it to Muriel, and spoke to her personally on the phone as soon as I was back in Glasgow.

There was a curious postscript to this affair. Pat, Robert's sister was putting her coat on to leave her house in Surrey to travel to Devon and give her mother the news of her brother's death when the phone rang. It was Muriel, who was ringing to give her the bad news.

"But Mum how did you know? Who told you? I was only told myself an hour ago."

"A man phoned from Truro. He said he was a clergyman from Sierra-Leone who had a cousin that worked in the British High Commission offices and was related to Cyril. You remember he was the horrible man who stole my things when I was ill in Robert's house. What he wanted I don't know. He pretended to give me his family's condolences but I put the phone down. I didn't know what to think, I didn't even know whether it was true. . . " Muriel was very distressed and her grief had not been helped by this gratuitous interference with the carefully thought out plans of Home Office, police and daughter to help her come to terms with Robert's death, when Pat should have been present to support her. In the middle of these anxieties and the sadness associated with my impending departure, it was good to have one's spirits lifted by the kindness and affection of my friends and colleagues, especially those I worked with at Marie-Stopes. Sylvia arranged a splendid party to which not only all the Marie-Stopes staff were invited but also my particular friends amongst the 'ex-pats', Ken and Kelly Shepherd, Hilary and Tom Cope, Richard and Isabelle Stowell, David Emery and his wife, and Maureen from the British High Commission and, of course Leona. Some friends had gone home before me but they had all filled the past months with such generous hospitality and kindliness that I found it difficult to realise that it was nearly a year since I had first arrived in West Africa.

All the staff, except May who had gone to a Marie-Stopes up-dating course in Kenya, with all she would need in my second-best suit case, were gathered in the unpretentious office and clinic accommodation at Adelaide Street for the farewell party – Admiya and Nancy, Mamie and Lauretta, Rebecca and Olive, Zaina and Keturah, Isata and Catherine, Marjorie and Regina, Alice and Fanta, Sister Cline and Sister Meux, Mr Mason (the accountant), the two recent medical recruits from Liberia and, warmly welcoming us all, Sylvia, the mistress of ceremonies. Many of the Sierra-Leonians were proudly arrayed in beautifully made local costumes of printed cottons in yellow and black, orange, yellow and blue, green and gold and combinations of colours which sound hideous but were brilliantly successful. Many embarrassing speeches were made and I was given a wonderful selection of personal gifts, from Sierra-Leonian anti-macassers to three beautifully embroidered dresses for special occasions with headscarves and slippers to match. These presents occupied almost all the space in my third-best suitcase and I treasure them dearly, although I confess that the two stones I had lost while I was in Africa was not long in returning and my special dresses remain in my wardrobe, unworn for two years.

After the formal speeches were over, everyone relaxed and the office staff miraculously produced plates laden with a typical Afro-European mix of good things to eat and plenty of Star beer and 7-Up to lubricate our palates and replace some of the perspiration. We were all beginning to suffer a little with so many in a relatively small space. The evening ended with dancing, no African party would be considered a party without it. Even I, totally unrhythmical as I am, was drawn into the conga and then I thankfully sank onto a chair and watched. The beat must be in the African genes. Sister Cline, short and stout, but so light on her feet she could have been a 'willie' from *Swanlake*, Isata, the epitome of all that is happy and joyful in these Sierra-Leonian people, and Keturah, the proud and dignified, laughingly pulling me back into the circle,

"You can't give up yet, Doctah Wilson!"

During the ten months I lived in West African I was never tempted to think in those terms but the practical difficulties of daily living, especially since I had been unable to drive, had made me look forward to returning to the colder, greyer skies of Glasgow. I was leaving behind me friends and colleagues whose warmth and kindness would never be replicated and with many of whom I am still in touch.

I have no illusions about 'doing good', I learnt as much about life and humanity as I taught about contraception. I have little faith in the long-term effects of Western involvement in Africa but Marie-Stopes Sierra-Leone needed a doctor in 1990 and I was available. One can only do the work in front of one on a day to day basis, each patient deserves one's whole attention and skill. If this unspoken message is transmitted to the staff with whom one works then, in a sense, one leaves a legacy. But in the chaos of post-colonial Africa, that inheritance is fragile indeed.

SIERRA-LEONE

HISTORY

1787	300 freed British slaves
1792	1100 freed Nova Scotian slaves
1808	British colony – Freetown area
1896	British protectorate – hinterland
1961	Independence
1971	Republic
1978	One party state
1992	Military coup (benign)

GEOGRAPHY

Tropical Climate

Hot (27.5)	Humid (3500 mrpa)
Dry season	December-April
Wet season	May-November

Resources

Agriculture	Minerals
Rice	Diamonds
Cocoa	Gold
Coffee	Bauxite
Palm Oil	Iron Ore
Ground Nuts	Rutile (titanium)
Cattle etc.	Chrome
Coffee	
Ground Nuts	

DEMOGRAPHY (1990)

Population	4.5 million approx
Population growth rate	2.7% p.a.
Fertility rate	6.5 births per woman of reproductive age
Child mortality rate	366/1000 by 5 years
Population under 15 years	Nearly 50%
Average age at first pregnancy	16 years
Maternal mortality	1000 women in Freetown in 1 year
Infant mortality	154 per 1000
Life expectancy	42 years (male), 38 years (female)
Adult literacy	18%